Jan Pleshette h[...]
and complemen[...]
years. A professio[...]
busy practice with writing extensively on her subject areas for numerous magazines, notably *Here's
Health*, *She* and *Family Circle*, as well as contributing
to various radio programmes.

Her books include *Health On Your Plate*, which was
highly recommended by the British Holistic
Medical Association, *Cures That Work* and *Overcoming
Addictions*.

INSTANT ENERGY
BOOSTERS

JAN PLESHETTE

ORION

An Orion Paperback
First published in Great Britain in 2001 by
Orion Books Ltd,
Orion House, 5 Upper St Martin's Lane,
London WC2H 9EA

A CIP catalogue record for this book
is available from the British Library.

ISBN: 0 75282 634 4

Typeset at The Spartan Press Ltd,
Lymington, Hants

Printed and bound in Great Britain by
The Guernsey Press Co. Ltd, Guernsey, C.I.

CONTENTS

ACKNOWLEDGEMENTS

My thanks to the following: Beverley Martin, Director of the Marian Institute for Analytical Therapy and Healing in London, for her invaluable advice on the Depression and Fatigue chapter; and for their help with the case histories, my grateful thanks to: Dr I. P. Drysdale, Principal, and college lecturer Lawrence Kirk, British College of Naturopathy and Osteopathy; nutritionist Breda Gajsek of the Institute for Optimum Nutrition; medical herbalist Janet Hicks; acupuncturist Richard James; Dr Andrew Lockie and his assistant, Chris Donne; medical herbalist Trudy Norris; Dr David Peters; medical herbalist Laura Stannard; and finally the Yoga Therapy Centre in London.

We all feel tired from time to time, when our energy runs low; after a long bout of work which has to be finished on schedule, a tremendous physical effort, or even an emotional experience (such as your own or your child's wedding). On these occasions we feel a natural tiredness, which disappears after a few early nights or a short break.

This book, however, is written for the person who finds that fatigue – from slight tiredness to an almost crippling exhaustion – is a persistent, nagging problem which, even with rest and a change, refuses to go away.

Fatigue has many causes. This book sets out to identify what's making you tired and offers self-help strategies to help you put matters right.

Constant tiredness is a ball and chain dragging you down. Unshackle yourself and find the abundant energy you need to get on with your life.

WHAT IS FATIGUE?

Fatigue is a burden, a bone-weariness that weighs you down all day, from the time when you crawl unwillingly out of bed, through a day when you try to cope in spite of heavy body and fogged mind, to the time when you collapse back into bed at last and try, probably unsuccessfully, to sleep.

Every day, at least one person goes to the doctor

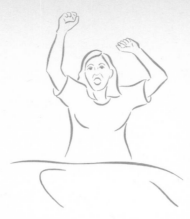

complaining of fatigue. In the US, almost one quarter of all the people in doctors' surgeries are there because they feel tired. In Denmark the figures are even higher: 41 per cent of women and 25 per cent of men.

There must be many thousands of others who don't want to bother their doctors about their fatigue. People hope that their tiredness will go away, perhaps tomorrow, or next month, or when the summer sunshine comes. But – too often – it doesn't.

> *Every day, at least one person goes to the doctor complaining of fatigue*

This book begins with Instant Energy in Four Simple Steps – quick ways to banish temporary fatigue which will work almost at once.

The Energising Break tells you how to recover your vitality and enthusiasm with a carefully planned twenty-four-hour break. The juice and fruit fasts can also be used long-term against ageing and overweight.

Nutrition is crucial. The Food and Energy chapter tells you how good food can give you energy, which foods take it away, and all about the supplements that can help you regain your natural vitality and health.

Some illnesses bring fatigue with them; see the Tired Body chapter to find out if any of these conditions apply to you, and what you can do about it.

Severe, continuous stress robs you of energy, leaving you so tired you can hardly think, let alone function properly. For many of us, stress is a habit, a way of life, something we're so used to that we don't even notice it any more.

Read the chapter on Stress and Fatigue and learn how to spot the stressors in your life and change your reaction to them through relaxation.

Depression is a lack of zest, when feelings of worthlessness, guilt and anger combine with profound fatigue. Depression is increasingly common nowadays, and much of it can be lessened or even cured altogether with self-knowledge and self-help. The Depression and Fatigue chapter outlines ways of emerging from this destructive and isolating state.

The health benefits of natural light and water have been understood by naturopaths for centuries. In Energy from Nature, find out how to get rid of midwinter blues with natural light, and actually increase your energy and vitality by simply using water from your taps.

As well as the yearly rhythms of summer sunshine, shortening autumn days, the dark winter and the rebirth of spring, our lives move in other cycles – monthly and even daily swings which cause our energies to fluctuate as well. By being aware of these body rhythms you can organise your life to make the most of your energy peaks and allow for your energy troughs: see Chapter 13.

Exercise creates energy

Exercise creates energy. The kind of exercise that you enjoy will fire you with optimism and well-being. In Energising Exercise, find out why this can happen, and how best to give your body the exercise it needs.

Most of us spend our working lives in unnatural environments. See the chapter Energy and Your Job to find out what is going wrong at work and what you can do about it.

Are you addicted to your work? Is your job sapping your strength so much that fatigue, hurry and anxiety have become a natural part of your day? In Work Addiction, discover if – and even why – you are a workaholic, and how to move towards a way of working that is better for you.

Your home is your refuge, a place where you relax. In Energy and Your Home, read about simple and inexpensive ways to make the place where you live a peaceful source of vitality and strength.

Finally, the five case histories tell the personal stories of people who have recovered from fatigue through complementary medicine and who owe their energy and good health to this flourishing branch of modern therapy.

CHAPTER 1

Instant Energy in Four Simple Steps

This chapter offers four ways to boost flagging energies when you need quick results. Going through these four steps will take you between five and a half and nine minutes.

Find a quiet place, free from interruptions, and follow the sequence without haste. If you haven't the time for everything, it's better to choose just one step rather than rush through the whole lot at top speed.

STEP ONE: GUARANA

Take two 500mg tablets of guarana with water, preferably on an empty stomach.

Background

Widely available in health food stores and pharmacies, the Brazilian herb guarana is a gentle stimulant which staves off fatigue. For more information, see Guarana in Chapter 4, Bonus Supplements.

STEP TWO: YOGA BREATHING

Good breathing – particularly yoga breathing or pranayama – acts instantly to dissolve tension and create energy.

Sit comfortably, or kneel, with your back straight. Throughout this exercise, breathe slowly and

> *Good breathing acts instantly to dissolve tension and create energy*

evenly, letting your breathing happen by itself, and pause briefly after breathing in or out.

1. Place your hand on your waistband so that it will rise and fall very slightly as you breathe in and out, gently and without strain, from the stomach. Once.
2. Place your palms on the sides of your chest and continue to breathe, but this time breathe in by expanding your ribcage only. Your hands are there to help you feel your ribcage expand and to press gently on it when you breathe out. Once.
3. Place your hand on your upper chest, just below the throat, and breathe in and out a third time, using the upper chest only. Once.
4. Finally combine all three in one long, revitalising in-breath – i.e. breathe in using the stomach; then, without breathing out, take some more air in by expanding your ribs; then (again without breathing out) finish your long in-breath by expanding the upper chest. Pause and now breathe out completely in three stages, starting with the upper chest, then the ribcage and ending with the stomach area.

Go through this calming and energising sequence once or more.

Time: Up to one minute.

Background

Yoga, one of several ancient paths to enlightenment and self-realisation, originated in the Vedas, scriptures sacred to Hindus which were first recorded between 1000 and 3000 BC.

The benefits of yoga as a system of exercise include greater calm, stamina and energy, with improved physical, emotional and psychological health. (For more on yoga, see Jason's case history in Chapter 2 and Chapter 14 on Energising Exercise.)

Pranayama means control of the prana, or life force, and is vitally important in hatha yoga. It enhances and harmonises energy flow.

My source for this exercise is *Yoga for Common Ailments* by Dr R. Nagarathna, Dr H. R. Nagendra and Dr Robin Monro (Gaia Books).

STEP THREE: ACUPRESSURE

Third eye point

This exercise relaxes, energises, clears the mind and banishes headaches.

Find the point between the eyebrows, in the hollow where the top of the nose joins the forehead.

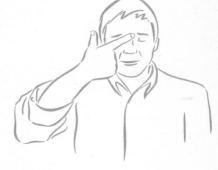

Press firmly with finger or thumb, applying pressure at a slight angle, for up to three minutes. If your hand gets tired, release the pressure for a few moments and then apply it again.

Sea of energy

This exercise relaxes, gives energy and strength.

Find the point three finger-widths below your navel, and press it firmly – your middle finger will probably be best – for up to three minutes, resting your hand from time to time if it gets tired.

Time: Up to six minutes unless you press both points at once!

Background
The ancient healing art of acupressure is related to acupuncture and uses pressure points on the skin to stimulate the body's inherent ability to heal and balance itself. Unlike needle acupuncture, however, acupressure is ideal for self-treatment because the points are easy to find and you simply use your hands.

My source for these exercises is *Acupressure: How to Cure Common Ailments the Natural Way* by Michael Reed Gach (Piatkus, 1995).

STEP FOUR: WATER

Run a cold bath and step into it (it's only for a few seconds and it's marvellously revitalising!); immerse your body up to the waist and stay there for about thirty seconds, with your feet propped up on the end of the bath. Get out and rub yourself dry vigorously.

Do not take cold baths if you:
• are menstruating
• are exhausted
• have just eaten a meal
• have a heart, blood pressure, breathing or circulatory condition
• suffer from thrombosis

Time: About one and a half minutes.

Cold water is terrific for clearing your head and giving you instant vitality

Background
Cold water is terrific for clearing your head and giving you instant vitality.

For more about water and health, see Water in Energy from Nature.

CHAPTER 2

Case History 1: Jason

J ason, aged thirty, is now a yoga teacher living in North London.

'About ten years ago I began to get very tired, mostly because of stress. I was sleeping a lot and was very lethargic; I felt a lot of tension round the shoulders and neck and my face felt tight. Even my eyes were affected; they felt tired. I was often cold, with poor circulation, and quite depressed.

'At that time I was in the States, studying at the University of Virginia and working as a waiter too. I developed back trouble, so I finally went to an osteopath.'

Jason found the treatments helpful.

'He gave me manipulation and showed me some exercises – yoga poses actually. He felt that my fatigue was caused by muscular tension.

'I started to feel more energetic quite soon. I got quite a bit better, but I was still retaining some tension and I didn't really know how to get rid of it.'

Back in London, Jason tried yoga classes, but the next real breakthrough came with a working trip to India.

'I heard about kundalini yoga. I was a bit sceptical at first; I knew that it was concerned with energy and that you needed a very good teacher. I happened to find a teacher who was marvellous – a maths professor who had a very scientific approach to yoga – and I felt very comfortable in his presence.

'Kundalini yoga works a lot on the deeper energy level, through chakras and what they call the subtle body. Visualising, some postures, lots of breathing; a lot happens in the mind and you can feel the energy (prana) moving round the body. Working in this way finally freed up all my energies.'

Jason calls his yoga practice the 'eyes light up' factor. 'I do it for about half an hour every day; if I stop doing it I will regress again.

'About five years ago I felt my office work was not quite right – sitting in front of a computer didn't feel healthy and natural. Eventually I quit my job and took an intensive teacher training course in yoga; I work now at the Yoga Therapy Centre in London, in an NHS project and locally.'

Jason is a good example of someone who uses yoga as much more than a valuable exercise system:

'Yoga has completely changed my life. I need a lot less sleep, I eat mostly a vegetarian diet now. Generally, physically, emotionally and mentally, I feel much much healthier.

'I am not talking about religion, I am just talking about a very scientific methodical practice. Yoga can transform your life, but you have to do it every day, you have to have the discipline. My fatigue is a fraction of what it once was.'

CHAPTER 3

The Energising Break

H

ere's how to set aside a whole day to yourself to really unwind, recoup your energies and give yourself a health and beauty treatment into the bargain.

For this totally relaxing and effective break, you will need:
- Fruit or vegetable juice of your choice
- Bottled or filtered water
- A dry bath brush
- Essential oils of lavender, vetiver, rosemary and geranium and a bottle of carrier oil (olive, safflower or almond are good). If you haven't time to get oils, just use your favourite bath fragrance and body lotion
- A much-loved book or cassette, and your radio, the cat or whatever else you may need, within easy reach.
- TV is not relaxing, so try to give it a miss. Reserve some undemanding tasks for this day, like writing letters, perhaps, or giving yourself a manicure. Later on, you could take a short walk in the sun or just sit in the garden. Try to persuade your partner to have a relaxing day too!

STEP ONE: THE TWENTY-FOUR-HOUR FAST

Your energising day is built around a fast. But we need food to make energy. So what's the sense in going without food if we are tired? Surely fasting will make matters worse?

Fasting is the ideal way of giving your body a chance to spring-clean itself, and it's not as difficult as you might think. With regular, sensible fasting, ageing is slowed, illnesses can recede and you will enjoy heightened energies and a greater zest for life.

But are our bodies really polluted? Where do these toxins come from? And what effect do they have?

> *Fasting is the ideal way of giving your body a chance to spring-clean itself*

A TOXIC WORLD

Our health nowadays is subjected to much abuse, which saps vitality and creates fatigue:

- We eat food that has been processed and otherwise manipulated
- We take little exercise
- We face a lot of stress
- We live in a world increasingly polluted with environmental chemicals – exhaust fumes, household and industrial compounds, chemicals in our workplaces (see Chapter 15) and so on.

Many health experts believe that our modern way of living leads to a gradual poisoning of cells with a consequent lowering of health, and that accelerating the body's valiant efforts to throw off these poisons is an essential part of getting well and staying well.

In her book *Ageless Ageing* (Century Hutchinson), health guru Leslie Kenton writes: 'The healing, rejuvenating and regenerating effects of a fast come from its ability to eliminate toxic waste products from the body – sometimes wastes which have been stored in the cells and tissues for almost a lifetime.'

FASTING

Fasting has a long and honourable history; all the major religions have used it at some time or another and fasting for health was practised by the ancient Greeks even before the time of Hippocrates.

Fasting – emphatically – is not the same thing as starving. To fast is to abstain from food while your body has enough reserves both to keep going and to nourish vital tissues. Starving uses up your reserves so that eventually vital tissues have to be sacrificed to keep you alive.

> **Fasting is not the same thing as starving**

During a fast your body turns naturally to stored nutrients; water is the only thing you must have. It's just possible to survive for about forty days on nothing but water (but don't try it!).

So, ignore well-meaning friends who tell you that you will collapse at once if you miss even a single meal, let alone three...

WHAT HAPPENS DURING A FAST?

The first thing you will notice, after only a few hours, is weight loss. However, because losses during your first fast are probably just fluid, you should only believe your scales when you are eating normally again. Regular short fasts will, over time, gradually reduce your weight.

Fasters often experience an ecstatic 'high', when the world is shining and wonderful and anything is possible. You will feel boundless energy and optimism and will probably start making feverish plans for your limitless future; this euphoria is part of the detoxifying process.

Fasting is a rejuvenating beauty treatment, too. As the body seizes this opportunity to detoxify, you will look and feel younger; you will easily see this with your skin, which will be clearer and smoother, and your eyesight may be sharper; you may feel sexier, too!

Fasting is a good cure for colds and catarrh and is prescribed by naturopaths for a long list of illnesses, both acute and long-term.

WHO SHOULD NOT FAST?

All this sounds marvellous, and it is. However, do not fast if
you are:
- pregnant
- breast-feeding
- under severe stress
- exhausted, weak or depressed
- receiving drug treatment

Do not fast if you have:
- anaemia
- high or low blood pressure
- heart trouble
- gout
- gastric or duodenal ulcers
- diabetes
- cancer
- a disease of the kidneys, liver or nervous system

Very young children, teenagers and the elderly should not
fast.

HOW TO FAST

For greater vitality, a short fast of twenty-four hours is ideal.
(You can extend this to three days, but longer fasts need the
supervision of a qualified naturopath or nutritionally informed
doctor who understands fasting.)

What to drink
Many experienced fasters stick to just water. However, juice
tastes much better and is more stabilising, particularly if you
suffer from low blood sugar (see Tired Body).

Orange and grapefruit juices are rather acid, so avoid citrus fruit. Choose one juice for your day's fast from apple, grape, or vegetable juices, diluting it with bottled or filtered water. These juices contain vitamins, minerals and starches, with alkalis to counteract the over-acidity of an empty stomach, and their potassium and natural sugar help to sustain your energy.

The very best juices are those you press freshly yourself – ideally from fruit organically grown. If you want to buy your juices, make sure they are labelled 'pure juice' and don't be fooled by juice 'drinks', which can be high in sugar.

Start your fast day by sipping a glass of hot water (preferably bottled or filtered; you can easily heat it in a pan) with perhaps a slice of lemon for flavour.

Food

During the day you should avoid all food; drink only juice and water. (This means, of course, no coffee, tea, or cola drinks; because you are having a short rest from these stimulants you may feel lethargic, and find that your reaction to them is stronger on the following day.) During your fast you should drink at least two pints of liquid, preferably more.

The idea of not eating at all can be pretty alarming, but you will find that it's often easier than taking tiny portions and longing for more. During this fast day, the times that you usually reserve for meals will be occupied by relaxing and taking your ease – not forgetting your scrub, bath and massage (later in this chapter).

How will you feel?

You may find today that your concentration and energy will be slightly lower, but this is only temporary; because your reaction time and co-ordination may be affected, you should not drive a car.

You may feel colder than usual with a slight headache, and your tongue may be coated with white fuzz. This is quite normal and a sign that your body, freed from the task of digestion, is rapidly setting about cleansing itself.

Your bowel action may slow down, too. This is quite common during a short fast and is nothing to worry about. On the other hand you should find yourself urinating more than usual, as your kidneys process unwanted fluid.

Breaking your fast

Breaking your fast is just as important as the fast itself. The playwright George Bernard Shaw once said: 'Any fool can go on a fast, but it takes a wise man to break it properly.' Eating huge meals the next day is fattening and unwise.

Break your fast the following morning with a small breakfast of ripe, fresh fruit.

Apart from its invigorating effect on mind and body, fasting helps us to listen to our own bodies and realise that we need only eat when we are hungry and not just as a habit, a reward or a prop. By daring to go without food for even a short while, we learn to choose food more wisely and enjoy it more.

FRUIT DAYS

Another way to detoxify, if you can't spend the day relaxing at home, is to have a fruit fast where for one day all you have is fruit, fruit juice and water. This is not so drastic so you'll still be able to go to work. This fruit fast can include any fruits you like, but you may find that citrus fruits – oranges, satsumas, grapefruit and so on – don't mix well with other fruits, so eat a small amount of them separately. Grapes are particularly good for fasts.

> A fruit fast once a week is an excellent way to detoxify and enhance your health

Buy only ripe, preferably organically-grown, fruit, and wash it thoroughly.

A fruit fast once a week is an

excellent way to detoxify and enhance your health over time and it will help you to control your weight.

STEP TWO: DETOX AND RELAX IN YOUR BATH

DRY SKIN BRUSHING

To boost the elimination of wastes through the skin, dry skin brushing before a bath or shower is ideal. It takes only a minute or two and leaves your whole body glowing and refreshed.

Take a dry bath brush – preferably a long-handled bristle one, but a hemp glove or a loofah will do – and brush your body firmly, working always towards the heart. Brush up your legs from feet to hips, up your arms from hands to shoulders, and in circular movements across your stomach, buttocks and back (this last is where the long handle comes in). Be sure to brush thoroughly down your sides, where congestion and cellulite form easily, from just under the armpits to the hips. Leave out face, neck and breasts.

Dry skin brushing stimulates lymph drainage, helping the lymph system to expel more wastes into the bloodstream for eventual discharge from your body. The lymph system relies on exercise, muscle contraction and gravity to work properly so any stimulus is a welcome bonus.

YOUR BATH

To revive your energies, add five drops each of rosemary and geranium, stimulating essential oils, to a warm bath. Wash yourself all over with a flannel to continue the good work done by the skin brushing. For a relaxing bath add instead five drops of lavender oil, used since Roman times for its powerful calming effect.

You can stay in the bath for up to twenty minutes or so,

topping up the water from time to time to keep it pleasantly warm.

AFTER-BATH MASSAGE

Make your own massage oil by pouring two teaspoonfuls (10ml) of carrier oil – virgin olive oil is good – into a warmed saucer and adding ten drops of lavender oil. Store what you don't use in a stoppered glass bottle in the fridge.

Pour a little oil into your palm and rub your hands together to warm it. Massage it into your breasts and buttocks with circular movements.

Pour a little more oil into your hands, rub your solar plexus (just above the navel) anticlockwise six times, then stroke your stomach upwards with both hands.

With a little more oil, stroke up each arm from hand to shoulder and finally, adding the rest of the oil to your hands, stroke your legs upwards with strong sweeps from ankle to top of thigh.

Remove any excess oil with kitchen paper or a towel and settle yourself, comfortably wrapped, on your bed.

...AND RELAX

By now, you should feel very relaxed and you may even want to doze for a while. If you are really in need of a complete rest, take the phone off the hook or turn on the answering machine.

If you still haven't shed all your tensions and anxieties, you can do your own relaxing easily and immediately. You simply rest one hand so that it covers your navel and breathe in so that your stomach rises slightly and your hand with it. When you breathe out your hand will fall. Continue this for as long as you like, feeling your whole body gradually getting heavier and tight muscles easing. If you feel breathless or giddy, stop this diaphragmatic breathing and go back to your usual breathing pattern. (For more about relaxation, see Stress and Fatigue.)

ACUPRESSURE

Acupressure originated thousands of years ago and is ideal for self-treatment because you just use your own hands to press points on your body.

Simple to use when you're lying down, these two safe pressure points will rapidly dissipate tension and anxiety.

1. *Centre of Power*

This relieves irritability and emotional stress. (Do not use this point if you have a serious illness.)

Find the point midway between the base of your breastbone and navel. Press firmly with the middle finger for two minutes, releasing the pressure for a few seconds if your hand gets tired. (To be used only with an empty stomach, so it's all right on your fast day.)

2. *Sea of Tranquillity*

This eases tension and depression.

Find the centre of your breastbone again and measure three thumb-widths upwards. Press the point firmly for three minutes, relaxing the pressure for a moment if you need to.

The source for these exercises is *Acupressure: How to Cure Common Ailments the Natural Way* by Michael Reed Gach (Piatkus, 1995).

Your energising day is designed to:
- help your body discharge some of the toxins causing fatigue, premature ageing and ill-health
- relax you completely, mentally and physically
- give you a deep rest so that you can resume your life tomorrow with increased energy and enthusiasm

---

CHAPTER 4

Food and Energy

Food is fuel and, to give you plenty of energy, it needs to be four-star.

Good food is easy if you stick to a few simple principles, it's not ruinously expensive and it's delicious. It keeps you healthy and give you continuous, long-lasting vitality.

Food now is very different from what Grandmother used to make – and even more remote from what our primitive ancestors would eat. They probably lived on fruits, salad plants, nuts and seeds, picked and eaten straightaway, with some fish and the occasional meat treat. (They didn't eat much meat to begin with because they weren't very good at catching it.) They had the same digestive system, and probably the same nutritional needs, that we have today.

> *Additives put into foods can affect our health, and substandard health means substandard energy*

Fast-forward several thousand years, and here we are now: junk foods, convenience foods – canned, dried, frozen or heavily processed – even a few foods irradiated and genetically modified for our delight…

What does this mean in terms of energy? Well, processing food means taking some things out, and putting other things in. Unfortunately for us, most things that are taken out are the very nutrients we need for energy, strong nerves, a powerful immune system and so on. Not only that: the additives put into foods can affect our health, and substandard health means substandard energy.

You can see this with ordinary white bread. To make white flour, the wheatgerm (one of the best energy foods you can get) is carefully milled out of the wheat grain and over a dozen nutrients – including many energising B vitamins – drastically reduced. To keep the final loaf fresh and attractive, a whole battery of food chemicals is added, some of which can cause problems for health.

You can't avoid altogether this distortion of our food unless you live entirely on whole, organic produce, which is free from chemical interference and is better for you (but sometimes expensive and hard to track down). However, you can choose wisely, to safeguard your own health and vitality and your family's as well.

What is the best choice to make?
Your cereals should be unrefined – wholemeal bread and wholegrain breakfast foods, brown rice and pastas. Your protein (fish, meat, cheese, nuts, seeds, soya) should be as unprocessed as possible, your fruits raw and ripe, salads crisp and fresh, and vegetables briefly cooked. Healthy fats are found in nuts, seeds, green leaves, oily fish, unrefined 'cold-pressed' salad oils and unhydrogenated margarines. Eat only moderate amounts of butter, cheese and milk.

Now, let's get down to details…

Is your diet actually making you tired? Find out in Energy Eating, below, how to put matters right.

The section on Bonus Foods and Supplements tells you which foods offer the most nutritional value and why. Do you really need supplements? Find out which nutrients are most involved in creating energy and, if you need extra help, which supplements will be best for you.

ENERGY EATING: IS YOUR WAY OF EATING MAKING YOU TIRED?

If you rush out of the house in the morning on just a cup of sweet black coffee, you'll get an energy high followed, an hour or so later, by a drop; you'll tend to feel more lethargic after lunch, too.

If you eat a large lunch, especially with pasta and wine, you'll feel sleepy afterwards. A lot of salt in your meal can cause fluid retention and can displace an energy-vital mineral, magnesium. Mixing proteins (meat, cheese, fish, etc.) together at one meal overworks your liver, encouraging fatigue. And bolting your food in haste will send you back to work more tired than ever.

Another large meal at the end of the day will overtax your already protesting digestion; calories eaten late tend to be readily stored as fat, too. Unless you are used to it, coffee-drinking in the evening will keep you awake and therefore more likely to be tired the next day.

THE ENERGY FAKERS

Do you have to boost your energy several times a day with cups of coffee and sugary foods? Here's what happens when you flog your already drooping energies...

Coffee, tea and cola drinks all contain caffeine, a powerful, but temporary, stimulant. This phoney boost soon runs out of steam, leaving you more tired than you were before and longing for another cup. Too much caffeine is bad for your nerves and can make you tense and anxious. For a steady energy supply, two cups of filtered coffee or four cups of tea a day have to be your limit.

It seems natural to reach for a sweet cake or chocolate bar for energy. But these refined, sugary foods only give you a quick temporary lift, swiftly followed by a drop — not much good in the long run — and they don't have the nutrients you need to create real vitality, either. Remember: white sugar offers

> *Too much caffeine is bad for your nerves and can make you tense and anxious*

you nothing but a fat middle – so boot it out of your diet!

If you have real problems giving up sugary foods, or if you're really hooked on tea, coffee or cola, see Low Blood Sugar, in the Tired Body chapter.

ENERGY EATING: WHAT TO EAT AND WHY

Have a substantial **breakfast** to keep you more alert, energetic and emotionally stable throughout the day. Cereal or wholemeal toast with perhaps scrambled eggs are better than a heavy, fatty, breakfast.

Wholegrains provide B vitamins with protein and fibre for a slow, steady supply of energy. Add some delicious yogurt for more protein and a little fat. (Fat is burned off quickly in the morning; it also slows digestion for continuous energy.) Add fresh, raw fruit for a tasty, nourishing breakfast. Coffee or tea with food instead of on its own is less likely to cause energy swings, and the vitamin C in a glass of fresh orange juice will help you absorb the iron in the cereal.

Eat a light **lunch**. Minimise that early-afternoon slump with a lunch of salad or some lightly cooked vegetables, a little protein and a small helping of carbohydrate (jacket potato or bread), followed perhaps by a piece of fruit. It's natural for some people to need a brief relaxer after lunch with feet up and even a short nap. Or you could take a few minutes' walk in the open air to perk yourself up.

At **teatime**, have a snack if you feel peckish. Don't let yourself get ravenous in the hope that this will control your weight; you may simply overeat at the next meal. Have a small roll with your cup of tea, or a piece of fruit with some juice.

The traditional glass of milk is a soothing bedtime drink

For **supper**, a light meal helps to keep your weight down (being fat makes you tired), and is ten times easier to stick to if you've started the day with a good breakfast. The traditional glass of milk is a soothing bedtime drink.

...And lastly

Give yourself time to chew your food slowly and well. By encouraging the flow of saliva in your mouth, chewing starts the release of energy-producing B vitamins from your food. And, of course, sitting peacefully enjoying your meal does wonders for your nerves, too.

COPING STRATEGIES

Have to miss a meal? Don't get starving hungry and wobbly: take at least eight 500mg tablets of spirulina (see Bonus Supplements) with a large glass of juice, preferably about an hour before mealtime. Spirulina – a tiny water plant pressed into tablets – offers a complete range of nutrients, as well as helping to suppress hunger pangs and stabilise your blood sugar, so you'll feel less shaky.

A standing lunch? Not a good idea! But if you must eat standing up, have just a snack, say a salad or a sandwich with an apple, some juice and perhaps a small coffee. This way you can eat slowly and digest well. Those danish pastries and croissants look very tempting, but they're refined foods loaded with sugar and fat – not helpful for after-lunch alertness and stamina.

BONUS FOODS AND SUPPLEMENTS

In this section, find out about the main nutrients that give you energy, the foods you will find them in and the supplements you might need, together with the best energy-promoting herbs.

Who needs supplements? Not everyone. But for some of us,

the right extra help can make a huge difference to our vitality and enjoyment of life.

Is your energy constantly being drained by poor diet or by challenges and problems in your life? Then your body may need extra nourishment; you can find out about it here.

Everybody's different. It's been proved that some of us need higher amounts of nutrients to stay healthy than others; needs differ, widely or just a little, from one person to another. This section will give you information about what you may need yourself.

> *Energy that is not created naturally will eventually let you down – with a bump*

Always bear in mind that the nutritional supplements and herbal remedies described here can help your body create its own natural energy, but that it's unwise to use them constantly as stimulants. Burning the candle at both ends has to stop sometime, and energy that is not created naturally will eventually let you down – with a bump.

Drugs: Are you on long-term prescribed medication? Drugs can destroy nutrients in the body; consult a nutritionally informed doctor or a qualified nutritionist for advice.

NOTE

Whole foods will give you the complete range of nutrients for optimum energy and health, but described here are the substances most directly involved with energy production, and which are successfully used by medical practitioners to treat fatigue. The safe recommended doses are higher than those found in food, because fatigue – like any other health problem – can bring with it severe nutritional deficiencies which require higher doses to put them right. (Recommended Daily Amounts, or RDAs – now being replaced with RNI,

Reference Nutrient Intake – are only the minimum amounts needed to stay well, plus a little extra.) If you are in any doubt, consult a nutritionally informed doctor or a qualified nutritionist.

Warning: Herbs are powerful substances and, as a general rule, it's best not to combine a herbal remedy with a drug your doctor has prescribed for you unless you are told that the combination is safe, either by an informed doctor or a qualified medical herbalist. (For your nearest practitioner, call the National Institute of Medical Herbalists on 01392 426022, 56 Longbrook Street, Exeter, Devon EX4 6AH.) For a postal answer from a respected herbal supplier, write to: Janet Lane, Information Service, GR Lane Health Products Limited, Freepost, Sisson Road, Gloucester GL1 3QB.

USING THIS SECTION

Turn to the B Vitamins first in the Bonus Vitamins section and check through the deficiency signs. A strong B-complex is a good place to start. Combine it with easy-to-grow sprouted seeds and grains, listed in the Bonus Foods. A couple of months later, add any other listed Bonus Supplements that you feel you need, with possibly ginseng or guarana.

To reap the maximum benefits from your nutrition programme, keep it up for at least six months.

BONUS FOODS

LIVER

The best meat food – primitive hunters would give the liver to the chief and the steaks to the underlings. Liver is an excellent source of protein, iron, vitamin A and the B vitamins, with some energy-balancing chromium among its many other nutrients.

The safest kind of liver is lamb's – these animals, in general, accumulate fewer toxins in their livers from modern agrochemicals and drugs than intensively reared livestock. However, the Department of Health advises pregnant women to avoid liver altogether so, if you're expecting a baby, it's best to play safe and leave it out of your diet.

WHEATGERM

Wheatgerm is the most nutritious part of the wheat seed. It's left behind in wholemeal bread, but is milled out for white flour, finding its way eventually to a shelf in a health food store.

High in energy-giving B vitamins, wheatgerm has healthy oils with protein, vitamin E and some iron and zinc among its many nutrients. (It offers octacosanol, too, available as a separate supplement and valuable for strength, stamina and energy.) Sprinkle wheatgerm freely on cereals, omelettes and casseroles before serving; cooking will reduce its nutritional content.

Note: Some brands are stabilised and will keep for a while outside the fridge; check the packet. Wheatgerm may not be suitable for you if you are allergic to gluten.

RAW JUICES

Some years ago, twelve Swedish men aged between twenty and fifty walked fifty kilometres every day for ten days, living entirely on raw fruit and vegetable juices with bottled water, vitamins and minerals. They finished their marathon in excellent health and spirits – a little thinner, that's all…

> *Raw juices can be a great help in throwing off fatigue*

Raw juices have been used for years by complementary practitioners; because they contain the nutrients of the original plant food, they can be a great help in throwing off fatigue.

How to make an energising juice

Wash well and chop some fresh, raw watercress or spinach – preferably organically grown – and juice it. Mix one dessert-spoonful of the juice with five dessertspoonfuls of bottled or filtered water and sip it slowly. Store any remainder in the fridge. Repeat eight times a day for two weeks.

SPROUTED SEEDS AND GRAINS

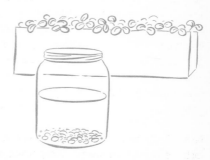

Here's a cheap, superbly nourishing food you can grow at home, even in a jam jar, using only water. These seeds take just a few days to germinate into tiny plants and, during this rapid sprouting process, huge quantities of nutrients are released to support their growth.

For the technically minded, oats when sprouted can increase their vitamin B_2 content by between 1300 and 2000 per cent, and their B vitamins – B_5, pantothenic acid, folic acid and biotin – by up to 600 per cent. The vitamin C in sprouted soya multiplies fivefold, and sprouted wheat's B vitamins go up by between 30 and 100 per cent, while its vitamin C goes up sixfold. Young sprouts contain easily digestible protein, plus essential fats and 'pacifarins', health-promoting agents found only in raw plant foods.

But before you rush out to the garden shed to bring in those left-over seeds, remember that ordinary sprayed seeds will dose with you chemicals, too, so always buy untreated seeds from a health food retailer, preferably date-stamped (after a year or so they are more reluctant to sprout). The most popular are mung, adzuki, soya and lentil beans; wheat, barley and oat grains; and pumpkin, sesame, sunflower, mustard, alfalfa and fenugreek seeds. (The sprouts from both tomato seeds and seed potatoes, however, are poisonous.)

How to grow them

Any suitable container will do – use an old jam jar or get a special plastic sprouter. Put in enough seeds to cover the bottom loosely, pour in plenty of water and leave them to soak overnight. The next morning, pour away the water (good for house plants) and rinse the seeds well, leaving them damp; a twice-daily rinsing will sprout them in a few days. To protect their flavour, keep them away from very bright light and extremes of temperature.

When they are just sprouting, and not yet plant-size, eat them raw as often as you like. They are deliciously crunchy sprinkled on hot soups, omelettes and casseroles just before serving, as a sandwich filling and, of course, as wonderful salad foods. Cooking destroys some of their nutrients, but if they have grown too long and spindly for raw eating, don't waste them altogether; soften them in boiling water for a few moments or stir-fry them briefly.

BONUS VITAMINS

THE B VITAMINS

Vital for energy, alert thinking and healthy digestion, the B vitamins work together as a team.

Best sources of vitamin B
* meats
* wholegrains, especially wheatgerm

- milk, eggs, cheese and yogurt
- pulses (peas, beans and lentils)
- green leafy vegetables and their juices
- fish
- sprouted seeds and grains

You're more likely to need extra B vitamins if:
- You are tired all the time and depressed, with a poor memory
- You have a poor appetite and are losing weight
- You are a heavy drinker
- You often get indigestion
- You sweat a lot
- You are taking prescribed medication (the Pill can cause a deficiency); ask your doctor
- You smoke
- You eat lots of foods made with white flour and white sugar

And… if you are a vegetarian or a vegan, you are more likely to lack vitamin B_{12}.

Dose: Take a good vitamin B-complex for up to six months for maximum benefits. If you get wind to start with, don't worry; it will wear off.

VITAMIN C

Gives widespread protection against fatigue, disease and ageing.

Best food sources of vitamin C
- all fresh raw fruits, especially citrus and soft fruits, papaya and tomatoes, and their juices
- all fresh raw vegetables, especially green peppers and watercress, and their juices
- sprouted seeds and grains

Dose: Vitamin C in the form of magnesium ascorbate or calcium ascorbate is better for sensitive stomachs; take 200 to 500mg a day with food for two months, reducing the dose when you start to feel better.

Note: Your body can get used to vitamin C, so it's not a good idea to stop it abruptly.

You're more likely to need extra vitamin C if:
- You bruise easily or have bleeding gums
- You get frequent colds and other infections you can't shake off
- You tire easily
- You smoke a lot
- You eat a diet low in fresh raw plant foods
- You take prescribed drugs; ask your doctor

VITAMIN E

Helps body cells and muscles make the most of their oxygen for energy, and improves circulation.

Best food sources of vitamin E
- wholegrain cereals, especially wheatgerm
- unrefined cold-pressed salad oils
- nuts
- eggs
- meat
- green leafy vegetables and their juices
- sprouted seeds and grains

Dose: Ways of measuring vary; take the top recommended manufacturer's dose with food daily for three months, reducing it when you feel better.

BONUS MINERALS

CHROMIUM

Chromium helps your body to use and store the blood sugar it gets from food, making sure you have a good steady supply of energy. It also helps to control your weight.

Best food sources of chromium
- egg yolk
- brewer's yeast (from your health food store)
- cheese
- liver
- wheatgerm
- wholegrain breads
- potatoes

Dose: Get Glucose Tolerance Factor (the best form of chromium) at your health food store and take 500mcg (micrograms) per day until you feel better.

Note: If you are diabetic, seek professional advice before taking chromium. If you are yeast-sensitive, choose another form of the mineral.

IRON

Among its many tasks, iron carries oxygen round the body to the muscles so they can work properly. Iron deficiency is very common, especially among menstruating women.

Best food sources of iron
- meat, especially liver
- fish
- wholegrain cereals, especially wheatgerm
- dried fruit
- molasses
- green leafy vegetables and their juices
- legumes
- nuts and seeds
- sprouted seeds and grains

Dose: Ask your doctor first before taking extra iron. With his or her approval, take 200mg of ferrous sulphate (the best kind) for six months, then cut the dose. Have some food, and a glass of orange juice, with the iron, for better absorption.

Iron deficiency is very common

You're more likely to need extra iron if:
- You are extremely tired all the time
- You have a pale skin and a sore tongue
- You get a hammering pulse after only a little exercise
- You have little appetite but suffer from indigestion
- You are depressed and confused
- You eat few salads and fruits (their vitamin C helps iron absorption)
- You are vegetarian or vegan
- You take prescribed drugs; ask your doctor
- You drinks lots of tea
- You add extra bran to your cereal or eat lots of chapatis

MAGNESIUM

Helps to keep energy high and nerves and muscles healthy.

You're more likely to need extra magnesium if:
- You are tired, depressed and irritable, with a poor memory
- You suffer from twitching muscles, or stabbing period pains
- You are a heavy drinker
- You add extra bran to your cereal
- You are often constipated
- You are on the Pill or other prescribed drugs; ask your doctor

Best food sources of magnesium
- wholegrain cereals, especially wheatgerm
- soybeans
- molasses
- green leafy vegetables and their juices
- milk
- nuts and seeds

- fish
- dried fruits
- sprouted seeds and grains

Dose: 200 to 400mg a day with food for three months; then reduce the dose.

POTASSIUM

Helps keep muscles and nerves healthy.

Best food sources of potassium
- wholegrains, especially wheatgerm
- nuts and seeds
- soybeans
- cooked red kidney beans
- lentils
- vegetables and their juices
- honey
- dates
- prunes
- fruits and their juices
- milk

Dose: 200mg daily with food for three months; then cut the dose.

> **You're more likely to need extra potassium if:**
> - You feel tired
> - You regularly take laxatives
> - You are a heavy drinker
> - You take prescribed drugs; ask your doctor

ZINC

Helps sustain energy levels and is necessary for good vision, resistance to illness and fertility.

Best food sources of zinc
- meat
- fish, especially shellfish
- lima beans, lentils and chickpeas
- green leafy vegetables and their juices
- wholegrains, especially wheatgerm
- soybeans
- cheese
- eggs
- seeds
- sprouted seeds and grains

Dose: Between 20 and 50mg a day with food for three months; then cut the dose.

You're more likely to need extra zinc if:
- You keep getting colds that you can't shake off
- Cuts and sores take a long time to heal
- You can't think straight
- You are depressed (especially after having a baby)
- You have white flecks on your nails
- You have lost your appetite, sense of smell, or sense of taste

---

BONUS SUPPLEMENTS
CO-ENZYME Q_{10}

You have Q_{10} in almost every cell in your body, where it helps to create energy. Without it, you'd be dead.

 Q_{10} is principally used to treat heart and gum disease, but its vital role in energy production has led to its growing use against fatigue and to enhance overall stamina. Some people are claiming other benefits, including better eyesight, stronger resistance to infection and even a better sex life.

Dose: Q_{10} is expensive and you need to take at least between 30 and 60mg a day for eight weeks to three months for results.

Note: The only known side effects have been slight indigestion in less than 1 per cent of those taking it. However, its safety for pregnant women has not yet been established. So, if you're expecting a baby, it's sensible not to take Q_{10}.

EVENING PRIMROSE OIL

Some people with severe fatigue have found evening primrose oil effective

This popular supplement is a rich source of Essential Fatty Acids, which – among other tasks – help the brain to work quickly and well. With a severe lack of EFAs, your body may misuse its blood sugar and you can get low blood sugar, making you feel ravenous and wobbly. EFAs, therefore, help to create energy, and some people with severe fatigue have found evening primrose oil effective.

Dose: 3g daily with food, spaced throughout the day, for at least three months; cut the dose when you feel better.

Note: You're more likely to need evening primrose oil if you suffer from PMS and have a dry, scaly skin. Do not take the oil if you are epileptic.

GINSENG

A herbal remedy used all over the world for thousands of years, ginseng is a shrub whose large, man-shaped root is known as the Root of Life. Cherokee Indians prized it so much that they would ask the earth's forgiveness every time they pulled up a plant.

Ginseng is traditionally used as an aphrodisiac, but modern research focuses on its effects on vitality, stamina and concentration. It is an 'adaptogen' – i.e., something that helps you to calm down or perk up when you need to, and generally deal better with stress. Russian astronauts chewed ginseng to help them cope with both the excitement and the risks of orbiting round the earth.

> *Ginseng is traditionally used as an aphrodisiac, but modern research focuses on its effects on vitality, stamina and concentration*

Siberian ginseng is a related newcomer; like the original herb it fights fatigue and stress but many experts believe it is safer. It is probably more suitable for women.

Brazilian ginseng or P*faffia*, a lush flowering plant from the rainforests, is a recent discovery. It is used by native Amazonians as a tonic and aphrodisiac and, again, may be especially suitable for women.

Dose for all ginsengs: Follow the stated dose for four weeks, leaving one week's gap before starting again. Give it a few months' rest from time to time; it's not a good idea to feel you can't do without a herbal remedy.

Note: Ginseng is not suitable for:
• pregnant women

- those with breast disease
- sufferers from high blood pressure

Some health freaks overdose on ginseng because it gives them a buzz. Don't; it can make you irritable and may have unwanted hormonal effects.

GUARANA

A flowering plant from the Amazonian rainforest, guarana has been used for centuries by natives to stave off fatigue, stimulate clear thinking and reduce appetite; it's also supposed to be an aphrodisiac.

Although guarana contains caffeine – about half that found in one cup of tea – it works gently and safely because other substances in the plant slow down and moderate the effects of the stimulant. Guarana helps you to stay energetic and calm for many hours, and offers a safe and effective antidote to fatigue.

The noted naturopath and author Michael Van Straten recommends guarana as a replacement for coffee for those who find that caffeine dependency is making them nervous and ill.

Dose: To begin with, take two 500mg capsules of guarana each day, first thing in the morning on an empty stomach. You should see the benefits after between seven and twenty-one days; then reduce the dose to one 500mg capsule a day, and keep going until you feel you can cope without it.

Note: Guarana has not been cleared for use by pregnant women. So, if you're expecting a baby, it's wise not to take it.

POLLEN

Pollen is gathered by the bees from flowers to feed their larvae. A complete food, it has all that humans need, too, in very small amounts and, over time, this team of nutrients can be an excellent tonic.

Pollen has long been used against fatigue and mental exhaustion; some athletes swear by it. It's easy to take for those who don't eat properly, and it can correct iron-deficiency anaemia. A special bonus is that, taken from January to August, it can lessen the misery of hay fever.

> *Pollen has long been used against fatigue and mental exhaustion*

Dose: One or two tablets first thing in the morning with a drink on an empty stomach; continue for at least three months to feel the benefits. (You can also get pollen granules to sprinkle on your breakfast cereal.)

Note: To start with you may notice an increased appetite – but this will soon wear off.

SPIRULINA

A form of algae growing in warm, alkaline fresh water, spirulina is 71 per cent protein, with almost all the B vitamins including B_{12}, many minerals, and high levels of both essential fatty acids and the health-giving pigment found in all plant foods, chlorophyll.

From the point of view of energy, spirulina's strength lies in its ability to prevent low blood sugar (see Tired Body, Low Blood Sugar) which can cause fatigue and confusion. For dieters, spirulina combines low calories with excellent nutritional value and its phenylalanine (an amino acid) content reduces the desire to eat.

Dose: Spirulina can initially encourage loose bowels – so start with low doses.

CHAPTER 5

Case History 2: Sally

London librarian Sally, twenty-eight, started feeling tired all the time a couple of years ago.

'I would wake up exhausted, having slept for hours, and I couldn't throw it off at all; at the end of the day I could barely get up the steps from the tube. I tried to keep up my body conditioning classes, but I stopped going – it was just too tiring, I had no energy for it any more. I wasn't going out much, just watching TV and falling into bed.'

Sally thought she might have candida, a common fungus-like condition which causes havoc in the digestive system and great fatigue, so she consulted a nutritionist and went on an anti-candida diet. But 'it didn't really help. I was eating a very healthy diet with lots of fruit and vegetables, and I took supplements, but none of it really worked, so I assumed I didn't have candida.

'I finally consulted Richard James, an acupuncturist in the same practice as my nutritionist. I actually went to him for something else – an ear infection – because I didn't want to take antibiotics. I told him about my fatigue.'

Sally responded at once to acupuncture. 'Richard took my pulses and looked at my tongue; he said my neck was causing the ear trouble and that my pulses were out of synch. He put some needles in, very briefly, on my wrists and various other points.

'After the first treatment, I felt transformed within about one day.'

Sally went back for another session with Richard James. 'I felt fine after that. Later on I went back again to Richard for irregular periods and other health problems. I also consulted an osteopath who immediately corrected the problem with my neck.

'My health is much better overall and my energy level is very good. I'm leading a normal life now – working very hard, socialising, exercising.

'I don't like needles at all,' Sally confesses, 'but I put up with them and it was worth it. I am told that I respond very well to acupuncture, and I would recommend it to anyone.'

CHAPTER 6

Tired Body

Here are nine common conditions which can make you tired. This chapter will help you to recognise if one of them might be responsible for your fatigue. However, if you are worried that it might be caused by a serious illness, you should consult your doctor (who will also be able to advise you if prescribed medication is depleting your energy).

IS AN ALLERGY MAKING YOU TIRED?

If you are allergic, your body is trigger-happy, overreacting to something that leaves most people unaffected, and giving you fatigue, stomach upsets, water retention, breathing problems, skin outbreaks and a host of other symptoms.

Allergens – the substances causing all the trouble – must be swallowed, breathed in or touched to have any effect. Common allergens are certain foods, petrol fumes, pollen, agricultural chemicals, the chlorine in swimming pools... But the complete list is almost endless.

What can you do if you think you have an allergy? Well, it's pretty obvious when you can't breathe every time you walk past a petrol pump, but a food allergy is harder to identify.

There are various tests that can pinpoint your allergens for you. If you think you have a food allergy (the commonest are to wheat and dairy foods), consult a qualified naturopath or nutritionist for help. You can even be addicted to a food you are allergic to (known as a 'masked allergy'), so the picture can be complicated.

An allergy is a sign of lowered vitality and, although drugs can control your reactions and you can take steps to avoid your allergen, the best long-term strategy is to concentrate on enhancing your well-being so that, with time, you may no longer be allergic.

> **An allergy is a sign of lowered vitality**

REMEDIES FOR ALLERGIES

A life with less stress and strain (see Chapter 8), exercise you enjoy (see Chapter 14) and an excellent way of eating (see Chapter 4) can do much to lessen or even cure your allergies.

- Your wholefood diet (minus, of course, any foods you are allergic to) should comprise plenty of fresh salads, fruits and vegetables (preferably organically grown) with protein and wholegrains.
- Cut out coffee, sugar, alcohol and all junk and convenience foods (some people are allergic to food additives).
- For super nutrition without a hint of chemicals, grow sprouting seeds and grains (see Chapter 4).
- Take small frequent meals so you don't get ravenous.

SUPPLEMENTS FOR ALLERGIES

Your practitioner will guide you; here, however, are some general suggestions:

- 1g of vitamin C can sometimes stop an allergic reaction within fifteen minutes.
- Pollen can fight fatigue and allergic hay fever (see Chapter 4).

- The herb ginkgo biloba can prevent allergic reactions; follow the stated dose.
- Quercetin, from water algae, can also stop allergic reactions; take 1 to 2g daily, with bromelain (found in pineapple).

ANAEMIA

The cells in your bloodstream that carry oxygen all round your body are constantly being renewed. The nutrients that keep this haemoglobin in good repair are mainly iron, vitamin B_{12} and folic acid. So, if there's a nutritional shortage, you will get anaemic.

ARE YOU ANAEMIC?

- Do you get out of breath with a hammering pulse after only a little exertion?
- Is your complexion pale?
- Do your ankles swell?
- Are the inside linings of your eyes pale instead of pink?

If you answer Yes to three or more of these questions, you could be anaemic and should see your doctor.

> **You're more likely to be anaemic if:**
> - You have heavy periods
> - You eat lots of bran
> - You are a vegetarian (you might lack vitamin B_{12})
> - You eat few vitamin C-rich foods – fruits, raw salads (vitamin C helps iron absorption)
> - You drink lots of tea or coffee

Ask your doctor to test you for possible deficiencies of iron, B_{12}, and folic acid.

REMEDIES FOR ANAEMIA

For foods and supplements to overcome anaemia see Chapter 4; liver, pollen, wheatgerm, iron and the B vitamins.

CONSTIPATION

Your bowels need to work regularly and well. Without this clearing of wastes from your body, you will feel tired and clogged up, with muddy skin, headaches and a greater risk of illness later in life. Laxatives flog the bowel and ultimately make it lazy; there's no substitute for the well-being that comes with natural, healthy elimination.

Because the colon needs bulk to push its wastes along, the best medicine for constipation is fibre, a natural part of our foods that we have been discarding for years. All that's necessary is to leave it in – and make sure you drink plenty of fluids to help it to work well.

THINK FIBRE

Think of fibre, and you usually think of wholemeal bread and wholegrain cereals with their bran naturally intact – or even bran on its own, added to foods. The dietary fibre naturally contained in wholegrains is fine, but the fibre in vegetables, fruits and salads is even better for both your bowels and your general health. Added bran can be abrasive for a sensitive stomach, and anyone

The skins and rinds of plants contain the most fibre. So, when possible, eat vegetables with their skins on

allergic to wheat won't be able to take it at all; it can also cause loss of minerals.

The skins and rinds of plants contain the most fibre. So, when possible, eat vegetables with their skins on – for instance, potatoes and carrots can simply be scrubbed – and your fruits unpeeled. The stalks of cabbage, broccoli and cauliflower contain plenty of fibre, too. Chew any fibrous foods well to make sure you absorb their B vitamins for healthy digestion, elimination and energy.

- Especially helpful are dried fruits, particularly figs and prunes.
- Some people find cider vinegar or yogurt useful, too. (Avoid UHT yogurt, whose beneficial bacteria have been wiped out.)
- Too much coffee or tea can constipate you; drink plenty of water.
- Stress can cause constipation and chronically unwilling bowels may reflect an emotional 'holding-back', so learn to relax. (See Chapter 8 for relaxation techniques.)
- Never put off going to the lavatory when you feel the need; unattended to, wastes simply retreat up the bowel again, making a movement more difficult next time.

REMEDY FOR CONSTIPATION

Cracked linseeds offer both bulk and healthy oils to get your colon working. Drink plenty of fluid first and add the linseeds to your breakfast cereal or yogurt, adjusting the dose to suit yourself. This wonderful medicinal food, which offers a host of health benefits, takes about seven days to work and should be continued indefinitely.

Exercise

Couch potatoes get constipated. Choose the exercise that you enjoy; stomach exercises are particularly good.

Complementary therapies

Reflexology, acupuncture and herbal medicine can help.

INSOMNIA

If you toss and turn for hours before sleep comes, you will find that daytime tiredness makes life very difficult.

Sleeping pills have side effects and are addictive so – except in an emergency – they are not the answer.

> *Creative, hard-working, rather introverted people tend to need more sleep*

But how much sleep do you really need? Some people can get by happily on fewer than eight hours. Creative, hard-working, rather introverted people tend to need more sleep; short sleepers can be extrovert and conformist. Which are you? Is it worrying about not sleeping that's really making you tired?

'I didn't sleep a wink last night,' some people say. The truth is they probably dozed off for a few hours, but weren't aware of it.

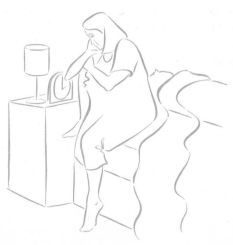

Do you habitually nap after lunch? The siesta is marvellous for revitalising you, but it cuts down on the sleep you need at night.

Why can't you sleep?
Commonest causes are:
- worry
- over-excitement
- over-tiredness
- lack of exercise
- indigestion
- bladder or prostate problems
- the later stages of pregnancy
- unfamiliar and disturbing surroundings

Smokers tend to take longer to fall asleep and some drugs can keep you awake; ask your doctor.

TIPS FOR BETTER SLEEP

1. Get up at the same time each morning, whether you've slept well or not.
2. Start to wind down several hours before bedtime, cutting out all demanding activities.
3. Sex is a good sleeping pill!
4. Don't drink coffee or tea later than 5 p.m.
5. Have a light snack half an hour before you go to bed; cheese and milk contain soothing calcium.
6. Run a warm bath, add a few drops of essential oil of lavender or clary sage and have a relaxing soak before bedtime.
7. Don't take your worries, resentments and fears to bed with you – talk them over if you can.
8. Open your bedroom windows and sprinkle a few drops of lavender or clary sage on your pillow for a relaxing fragrance.
9. If you are wakeful in the night, get up, walk around or read

a book for a few minutes, then plump up the pillows and go
back to bed again.
10. Most importantly, learn to relax; see the chapter on Stress
and Fatigue.

REMEDIES FOR INSOMNIA

Nutrition

100–150mg of calcium with 200–500mg of magnesium daily
with food.

Homeopathy
- For someone with mental strain who wakes around 5 a.m.,
then falls asleep again: Nux. Vom. 30c.
- For someone afraid of not sleeping, who gets nightmares:
Ignatia 30c.

Take one dose one hour before bedtime for ten nights; repeat
during the night if you wake up.

Note: Do not take homeopathic remedies within twenty
minutes of eating, drinking (except water) or using tooth-
paste: it prevents them from working effectively.

Herbal medicine
Valerian is proven to give better sleep. Take the recommend-
ed dose.
Camomile tea is very relaxing before bedtime.

Note: Use herbal sleeping remedies for a limited time only;
it's not a good idea to feel you can't do without them.

Complementary therapies
Reflexology and acupuncture can help.

LOW BLOOD SUGAR

Most people get temporary low blood sugar from time to time – an abrupt plunge in energy which leaves you feeling exhausted, ravenous and muddle-headed, but which soon wears off.

But frequent low blood sugar – or reactive hypoglycaemia – can be a real health problem, causing inexplicable bouts of fatigue and many other unpleasant symptoms.

DO YOU HAVE FREQUENT LOW BLOOD SUGAR?

- Do you feel tired when you wake in the mornings?
- Do you feel shaky when you are hungry, terrible if you miss a meal and more energetic after you've eaten?
- Do you often crave chocolates, sweet cakes and other sugary foods?
- Do you get an energy drop mid-morning or mid-afternoon?
- Do you have to drink coffee or tea all day just to keep going?

If you scored four or more, you probably have a low blood sugar problem.

WHAT IS LOW BLOOD SUGAR?

When we eat, the glucose, or blood sugar, circulating in the blood goes up. Normally, the pancreas releases insulin which brings the blood sugar down again. But if this mechanism isn't working properly, too much insulin is released, bringing the blood sugar down with a bump. Because the brain needs plenty of blood sugar to work properly, if levels fall too drastically we feel confused, irritable, hungry, headachy and tired.

What causes low blood sugar?

In vulnerable people, this see-saw effect can be triggered by:

- refined sugars and starches
- caffeine
- tobacco
- alcohol
- anything you are allergic to
- too much exercise or stress

Some drugs can cause low blood sugar; consult your doctor.

> *Because the brain needs plenty of blood sugar to work properly, if levels fall too drastically we feel confused, irritable, hungry, headachy and tired*

REMEDIES FOR LOW BLOOD SUGAR

- Cut out the triggers listed above as much as you can.
- Cut out all added sugars, even honey, and don't drink fruit juice on its own without food.
- Take small frequent meals of unrefined foods (instead of large meals spaced further apart) so that you never get hungry.
- Have a small snack before going to bed, too; this could be crispbread and cottage cheese, a glass of milk and a whole-meal sandwich, or some yogurt and a little fruit.

Don't worry about putting on weight; you'll be eating the same amount of calories, simply spaced in a different way.

Supplements for low blood sugar

Spirulina helps to stabilise blood sugar, and a chromium supplement, over time, can help sugar cravings; see Chapter 4.

Consult a nutritionally informed doctor or a qualified nutritionist for more advice.

ME OR CFS (CHRONIC FATIGUE SYNDROME)

ME is like having a hangover, muscle pain and exhaustion from running a marathon, and brain fag all at the same time. This disabling condition can drag on for weeks, months, sometimes even years.

ME affects the immune system, the glands, the digestion and the brain – so you can have speech, vision and balance problems among its long list of possible symptoms.

WHAT CAUSES ME?

It often develops after a viral illness which you can't seem to recover from, or after long periods of severe stress or overwork, or it can be linked to allergies.

ME can strike anyone, but its victims are most likely to be fit, hard-working people aged between twenty and forty – which is why it used to be called Yuppie Flu.

If you think you may have ME the first thing to do is to ask for a laboratory test and diagnosis. Although there are no drugs specifically for ME, antidepressants sometimes help (but many drugs make people feel even worse). However, you can do a lot to help yourself.

Your main problem will probably be forgiving yourself for needing so much rest. Because symptoms shift around so much, and progress seems to be 'two steps forward and one step back', you're likely to be depressed and frustrated, impatient to get better and live life to the full again. Dealing with these feelings, and developing great patience, are essential first steps.

Rest – to start with, a lot of rest – is vital to your progress and if you try to push yourself beyond your own current, very humble, limits you won't get any better. Exercise is good for ME sufferers, but only as much as you can do and no more; one of the main symptoms is extreme exhaustion after only the mildest exertion.

DIET

You may have food allergies or candida, and need to consult a nutritionally informed doctor or a qualified nutritionist. Apart from this, good general guidelines are:

- Cut out wheat, dairy foods, sugar, caffeine, alcohol, saturated fats, spices, salt, red meat and all junk foods (don't worry – there's plenty left to enjoy!)
- Stick to whole, unprocessed foods as much as possible, with plenty of raw salads and fruits if you can tolerate them.
- Sprout easy-to-grow seeds and grains for super nutritional value (see Chapter 4).
- Drink plenty of water – bottled or, better still, filtered (see Water).

Supplements for ME
Magnesium and Efamol Marine (or just evening primrose oil) can be helpful, and co-enzyme Q_{10} is often recommended. (For more information on the above, see Chapter 4.) The bee product, propolis, may also help.

Complementary therapies
Reflexology and homeopathy have been proved valuable. See Rosemary's case history in Chapter 7.

Yoga and osteopathy, to enhance all body functions, would help as well.

Relaxation

See the Stress and Fatigue chapter and learn to relax deeply for an important part of your recovery programme.

For more information

Valuable and comprehensive help is offered by Action for ME, PO Box 1302, Wells BA5 1YE. Call their twenty-four-hour helpline on 0891 122986, or visit their website at www.afme.org.uk.

OVERWEIGHT

Being fat makes you tired – as well as creating other health risks – because there's more weight for you to carry around.

Here's how to plan lifelong weight control in an intelligent way, without half-killing yourself with temporary fad diets which can make life very difficult.

The convenience foods you see advertised everywhere are loaded with fat and sugar and are high in fattening calories. This is, of course, bad news for your weight. But less well known is the fact that the appestat in your brain, which tells you when you have eaten enough, will not work properly unless it is nourished with whole, unprocessed foods. This means that, without this natural warning system, you will tend to overeat anyway.

Do you go on crash diets?   Then you'll know that, as soon as you go back to your original way of eating, you put all the lost weight back on again. Diets are useless because they are temporary. This also applies to slimming aids and, of course, to slimming drugs, which carry health risks as well.

Do you crave sweet things, even though they make you fat?   Refined, sugary foods give you a rapid rise in energy followed by a drop and more cravings. Chromium, an essential mineral found in egg yolk, brewer's yeast, cheese, liver, wheatgerm, wholegrain breads and potatoes, can reduce these cravings over time.

Do you crave any other foods? The foods you're most likely to be addicted to are coffee, dairy foods, eggs and wheat. As well as needing these foods every day, and craving them when they're absent, you can also be allergic to them, and this will cause you to retain water when you eat them – double trouble! For more about this, see Allergies.

Do you eat certain foods because of your mood? Because you're depressed, bored, anxious, or feel you deserve a reward? Are some foods what Mother used to make, and that's why you stick to them? Are you fat because you want to keep other people at arm's (or body's) length? Greater awareness of these powerful factors will help you plan your eating more effectively.

Do you avoid exercise? If you are overweight, you may be inactive because you have a heavier body. You may also be ashamed of your shape. (Remember, however, that in an exercise class everyone looks in the mirror at themselves, not at anyone else.)

SLIMMER FOR LIFE

You need foods that contain nutrients and fibre to give you a slow, steady supply of energy and an efficient appestat. Concentrate on:

- wholegrains
- protein
- fresh salads
- fruits
- vegetables (where possible with skins on) and their juices

- unrefined 'cold-pressed' salad oils (a lack of essential fatty acids in refined oils may cause ravenous hunger and you'll thus be worse off than ever)

Eat lightly later in the day for permanent weight control

Breakfast is vital and should be substantial; calories eaten early in the day are burned off as energy whilst calories eaten later tend to be stored as fat. So eat lightly later in the day for permanent weight control; ideally, have breakfast, lunch and a snack tea, and eat little or nothing at night. The occasional bar of chocolate or gooey treat will make little difference over time and, of course, you can't offend your dinner party hostess by nibbling on an apple and one lettuce leaf!

Chew everything and take your time. This gives your appestat a chance to signal Full Up so that you eat less, as well as treating your digestion more kindly.

Make the changes to this way of eating over several weeks; after all, it's for a lifetime.

Weight loss, after an initial drop, will probably level out for a while and it's better not to think in terms of rapid, dramatic results. This way of eating soon becomes a pleasant habit and you won't want to change back; your firmer figure and increased energy will show themselves in good time, and they will be with you to stay.

Exercise

Find something you enjoy and that fits into your lifestyle; start gently, and keep going. Exercise firms your body, uses up calories and makes you feel good into the bargain. See the chapter on Energising Exercise for more ideas.

Supplements to counteract overweight

A good vitamin B complex, with chromium, can help, as can spirulina before meals.

Co-enzyme Q$_{10}$ and evening primrose oil can both cause a slight weight loss in overweight people.

For more about all these supplements, see Chapter 4.

If you need more help, consult a qualified nutritionist or join a reputable weight-loss group.

PREMENSTRUAL SYNDROME

Do you suffer from tiredness, headaches and irritability, with weight gain, tender breasts and sugar cravings, before your period?

Then you are one of the 40 per cent of women who suffer from Premenstrual Syndrome.

The menstrual cycle is a very complex, delicately balanced hormonal process and most doctors now believe that PMS is mainly caused by hormonal imbalance.

Nutrition is vitally important for PMS and, over time, can work wonders:

DIET

Eat plenty of:
• fibre-rich whole cereals
• green leafy vegetables
• legumes
• fruits
• wheatgerm and lamb's liver for extra B vitamins
• fish

Limit your intake of:
• refined white sugar (which can cause energy switchbacks)
• salt
• red meat
• cheese
• alcohol

- coffee
- tea
- chocolate
- cola drinks

If you're a smoker, cut down!

If you have sugar cravings, which usually accompany severe fatigue, take small frequent meals of whole foods free of added sugar. For more advice, see Low Blood Sugar.

> *If you have sugar cravings, which usually accompany severe fatigue, take small frequent meals of whole foods free of added sugar*

Supplements for severe PMS

Throughout the month, take a strong vitamin B complex which gives you 100mg of vitamin B_6 per day (a proven safe dose) together with 500mg of vitamin C, 300mg of magnesium and 100IU of vitamin E daily, all with food.

For two weeks before your period, add three 500mg capsules of evening primrose oil daily, one with each meal.

Continue your food and supplement programme for at least three months to feel the benefit, then gradually reduce the supplement doses.

Instant helpers during PMS

Stock up with dandelion or nettle tea from your health food store to help your kidneys get rid of excess fluid (don't drink either after 5 p.m. or you'll be up all night running to the loo!) and get some camomile tea for a mild sedative.

For knife-like, cramping pains, dissolve four tiny tablets of Mag. Phos. (a biochemic tissue salt) on your tongue with sips of hot water every fifteen minutes or so until the pains ease.

Women who exercise suffer less from PMS

Exercise

Women who exercise suffer less from PMS. Even a gentle walk every day will help. See the chapter on Energising Exercise.

Relaxation

See the Stress and Fatigue chapter for relaxation that really works, and set aside a time every day for yourself.

Complementary therapies

PMS responds very well to reflexology and herbal medicine.

For more information

Contact the Women's Nutritional Advisory Service, PO Box 268, Lewes, Sussex BN7 2QN; directory helpline 09062 556615; website www.wnas.org.uk.

UNDERACTIVE THYROID

Your thyroid gland is a plum-sized lump in your neck just under the chin. It controls the speed at which your body works and how much energy you have. Underactive thyroid is particularly common in women (an overactive thyroid is comparatively rare).

A severely underactive thyroid is obvious from hospital tests and can be effectively treated with drugs. However, a slightly underactive thyroid, though it may not show up in tests, can still cause trouble.

DO YOU HAVE A SLIGHTLY UNDERACTIVE THYROID?

- Are you always tired?
- Do you feel the cold easily?
- Do you have great difficulty in losing weight?

- Are you often constipated?
- Do you have a dry skin with dry, thinning hair?
- Do you constantly have to urinate?
- Do you often get confused?

If you answer Yes to four or more of these questions, then you could have a slightly underactive thyroid and you should first of all consult your doctor.

If tests prove negative, and you are still not satisfied, here's how you can help yourself.

REMEDIES FOR UNDERACTIVE THYROID

- The thyroid needs iodine, so eat more iodine-rich foods – shellfish, saltwater fish, seaweed.
- Many table salts have added iodine.
- Do not add bran to your cereal.
- An underactive thyroid is made worse by smoking.
- Stress can upset the thyroid, but aerobic exercise helps it to work.

Complementary therapies

Consult a qualified nutritionist or naturopath for advice on nutrition and lifestyle. Homeopathy, medical herbalism, acupuncture and reflexology can all help.

Persistent thyroid problems need a comprehensive treatment programme from a skilled practitioner.

CHAPTER 7

Case History 3: Rosemary

Rosemary, twenty-six, is a speech therapist working in North London. Her fatigue first started in September 1997, when she got flu and couldn't shake it off.

'At the time I had just started college and I was working really hard. I was terribly tired all the time; I had joint and muscle pains, my eyes felt tired and my skin was very sensitive to touch. If I tried to exercise, I would feel absolutely prostrated with exhaustion afterwards.'

Rosemary's doctor did not initially diagnose her condition but gave her antidepressants which didn't help. Meanwhile, she tried to keep up with her studies.

'In the end my mother persuaded me to go to Dr Lockie in Guildford for homeopathy. Dr Lockie diagnosed ME. He gave me homeopathic medicine, with advice on diet, and supplements.'

Rosemary saw Dr Lockie about once every couple of months over the next three years.

'I gradually began to notice changes for the better. As I improved, he would change the homeopathic remedies to suit my changing state.

'I seldom have junk foods, caffeine or refined sugar, and I eat very little wheat. I have goat's milk and soya. I have been vegetarian for several years anyway.'

Rosemary finally qualified and left college, but didn't start work straightaway. 'I was still at the stage where, if I got an infection, I would feel absolutely zonked, so I took six months off.

'During this time, I saw a healer who gave me hands-on healing for half an hour daily over six days, and that boosted my energy levels tremendously; I felt so much better afterwards. The effects have lasted ever since. If I get run down and tired again I go back to Dr Lockie and the healer and they put me right.

'What can I do now that I couldn't do before? Almost everything! I work hard, I walk and swim a lot, I feel a new person. My energy now is very stable, without ups and downs. But I still need plenty of sleep and, if I get an infection, I am always very careful to recover completely before going back to work again. In some ways I feel my health is better than it was before I got ME.

'I would recommend homeopathy and/or healing for anyone with ME for gentle holistic benefits without side effects. Different things work for different people – listen to your body for which therapy feels right for you.'

CHAPTER 8

Stress and Fatigue

Stress and strain are everywhere nowadays and, for many of us, fatigue caused by stress is a permanent part of life. In balancing the demands of work, home and relationships, it often seems that there's no let-up. Trying to cope with all this can drain our energies in a vicious circle that leaves us less and less able to deal happily and effectively with our lives.

> *Fatigue caused by stress is a permanent part of life*

WHAT IS YOUR LEVEL OF STRESS?

To find out your stress levels, answer the following questions:

- Do you often feel so tired you can't even think any more?
- Do you hurry all the time, even when there's no need?
- If someone bangs a door, do you jump?
- Do you lie awake at night, mulling things over?
- If you get the chance to rest in the daytime, do you find it impossible to doze off?
- If you have to deal with a difficult situation, do you suffer from any of the following: pounding heart; damp palms or very cold hands; frequent urination; rapid, shallow breathing; a tight band across the midriff so you can hardly breathe?
- When you are extremely overworked, do you find it difficult or impossible to slow down?

- Do you cry or lose your temper at the least thing?
- Do you get depressed, with headaches, insomnia, constipation or indigestion?
- Do you dread Mondays and work?
- Do you come home knowing that yet more problems are waiting for you?

If your answer is Yes to more than two of these questions, you are carrying a burden of stress. If you answer Yes to all of them, you are running the risk of damaging your health.

Stress makes you tired, of course. But it can also make you ill; stress-related disorders include high blood pressure, heart disease, migraine and many other conditions – and it can even kill, just as surely as a well-aimed bullet.

So, to beat stress, you first need to understand how it affects you.

WHAT IS STRESS?

How does stress damage us? And what exactly is it?

Strictly speaking, stress is any change which demands an adaptation, an effective response, from us.

Stress is often exhilarating. The intense concentration and flat-out effort of the athlete or dancer; the marvellous high when you've come through a tough exam with flying colours; coming home from a new job knowing that, after the first few hectic days, you enjoy it and can cope with it: who would be without these challenges?

But – imagine you are stuck in a long queue of cars, inching forward with painful slowness, while on the pavement little old ladies, toddlers and snails flash past. You are going to miss that flight... Or, you're peacefully decorating your new flat, and there's a peremptory ring at the door. 'Come in,' you say through gritted teeth to the critical mother-in-law/difficult maiden aunt/impossible friend with man-eating dog on the doorstep. All these experiences – both pleasant and unpleasant – call for adaptations from you and therefore come under the heading of stress.

FIGHT OR FLIGHT

To understand how our bodies react to stress, we need to go back to the time when we were just one animal among others, living in the open with danger always around the corner. When these primitive people were threatened it was a matter of life or death to be able to get away in time. They had to be quick enough to catch their prey, too, and resourceful enough to defend tree or cave against invaders. So, in an emergency, they needed instant speed, stamina and quick thinking.

The built-in body changes that helped these early people to survive are with us now, and they are called the Fight or Flight Response. (The body reacts, in fact, to any kind of stress, pleasant or unpleasant, in the same way.) Hormones respond immediately, causing both the instant release of extra energy and faster mental reactions; blood pressure goes up to push more nutrients into the tissues; and breathing and heart rate quicken, giving a better turn of speed, which is further helped by an increased blood supply to arms and legs. After the crisis and its demands are over, the body sets about repairing itself, exhaustion takes over and we need to rest.

Nowadays, life doesn't usually involve hunting for live food or shinning up a tree pursued by wolves. But if we are stuck in that traffic jam, or confronted with those terrible relatives, the body reacts in the same primitive way.

The difference is that this Fight or Flight Response can be inappropriate in the modern world. A few minutes' patience and a traffic jam usually clears, and a smile with some tactful words usually deals effectively with unwanted visitors.

So, our stressors are different now. In an uncertain, rapidly changing world we need, not to be able to fight back with club

> *Usually, it's not so much the actual stress that causes trouble; it's our inability to deal effectively with it*

and rock, but to cope calmly, to use our energies wisely, to be able to relax. Usually, it's not so much the actual stress that causes the trouble; it's our inability to deal effectively with it. We need, not brute force, but patience, coolness and flexibility.

All this is in your own hands. For you can decide for yourself how you are going to deal with stress. You can decide to react to the irritations and frustrations in your daily life in a different, calmer way, reserving your energies for more pleasant activities.

How do you deal with stress?

Fred arrives home dishevelled and furious (though he is only a little late), grumbling because it's raining and insisting that his evening is ruined because the cat has been sick again.

Harry was in the same slow train but, instead of fruitlessly getting in a state, he read his paper. A little rain hurts no one, thinks Harry, and a bowl of water will soon sort out the mess left by Tiddles.

Fred is exhausted, but Harry is ready to go out with his girlfriend… The same situation – but two widely different reactions.

RELAXATION

The quickest and most effective way to change your response to stress is to relax. If you know how to relax, you can use simple daily techniques to make your day easier and much more pleasant. To be able to calm yourself whenever you need to is a formidable weapon against stress which, practised over time, will help you to become a more peaceful and energetic person.

Forget the tranquillisers; the power can come from within yourself.

GOOD BREATHING

First, learning to relax involves learning how to breathe calmly and well – after all, you did it when you were a baby.

Breathing is something we take for granted. But all our body functions are affected by the way we breathe. By altering your breathing, you can quickly calm your nerves and relieve strain and anxiety.

Good breathing is an essential part of relaxation techniques; over half a century ago, medical researcher Eric Strauss was using breathing exercises as a treatment for emotional tension. Our disharmony with ourselves, our fears and worries – all are profoundly influenced by the way we breathe.

What happens when we breathe?

Your lungs are protected by twelve pairs of ribs and the two lowest pairs, just above the waist, are 'floating'; unlike the others, they are not fixed to the front of your chest. This means that the lower parts of your lungs have more room to expand in than the upper parts. This expansion is made even greater by the diaphragm, a dome-shaped muscle just below the floating ribs, which rises and falls when you breathe in and out.

A sensitive mirror of your feelings, the diaphragm tightens to reflect tension, and the solar plexus – at the mid-point of the diaphragm just above the navel – is a veritable storehouse for your feelings, reacting to every change of mood. Because the diaphragm's movements account for about two-thirds of the lungs' expansive capacity, any tightness and rigidity stored there will have a huge effect on how you breathe and how much air you can take in. Equally, diaphragmatic breathing eases all this stored tension and helps you unwind.

Good breathing not only revitalises and relaxes, it massages your digestive system and even helps the heart to work better, too.

Partly because of its calming effect, and partly because taking deep breaths is one of the pleasures of smoking, many smokers find that good breathing can help them to kick the habit. Some dieters, too, find that its soothing effect helps by subduing a nervous desire to eat.

Bad breathing – common not only in tense people, but also in those with lung disease – allows stale air to linger in the lungs, creating a breeding ground for germs and a hindrance to your body's oxygen supply.

So, here's how to breathe naturally and well – just like you did when you were in nappies, in fact.

RELAXING IN TEN SECONDS

Until you get the feel of this exercise, lie comfortably on a bed or on the floor with one hand resting on the centre of your waistband.

You are going to breathe in a way that is perfectly natural and easy, but which over the years you may have forgotten. Breathing should not be a strenuous, effortful process; it's just something that usually happens automatically, so never think of gulping in deep breaths and trying hard. As you breathe gently, become aware that your hand is rising slightly each time you inhale and going down again every time you exhale. It's a very slight movement and you'll hardly notice it.

(Some people find this way of breathing very strange and awkward to start with, but that's because they haven't done it for a long time. If at any time you feel headachy, tense or out of breath, stop and go back to your ordinary way of breathing; you can try again later.)

When diaphragmatic breathing comes easily to you, add one other thing. Every time you breathe out, think of every part of your body getting heavy in turn – shoulders, arms and hands, stomach, hips, legs and feet. Feel the heaviness on each out-breath weighing you further down so that, very soon, you will be completely relaxed.

Once you can do this exercise easily, you can use it anywhere without your hand, sitting, standing or even walking along, and, of course, it's invisible! A few seconds of this tranquillising breathing will wash away your tensions and stress and make your day much easier.

> A *few seconds of tranquillising breathing will wash away your tensions and stress*

RELAXING IN FIVE MINUTES

As soon as diaphragmatic breathing comes naturally, you can go a step further.

All you need for deeper relaxation is an easy chair or a bed and five minutes to spare. Make yourself really comfortable.

You're going to use an adaptation of Autogenics (AT), a proven method of relaxation. Continue diaphragmatic breathing throughout; you shouldn't have to think about it by now.

You're going to repeat six phrases silently to yourself; to start with, of course, you'll have to keep this book by you until you know them by heart.

These phrases are designed to cause a response of increasing relaxation from you. You don't need to worry about AT's effectiveness – it will work, whether you think it's going to or not.

Repeat each one of the following suggestions silently to yourself three times, without haste:

• 'My right arm is heavy.'
• 'My arms and legs are heavy and warm.'

- 'My neck and shoulders are heavy.'
- 'My back is broad and soft.'
- 'My whole body is relaxed.'
- 'I am calm.'

(Note that, if you are left-handed, you need to begin with 'My left arm is heavy' instead.)

This takes a couple of minutes. You can if you wish repeat the sequence, or you can just lie in a peaceful state until your five minutes are up.

When you get up, clasp your hands firmly together to rouse yourself and get your energies flowing again.

You can practise this marvellously calming and energising sequence once a day or more; it's a boon when you go to bed or before a situation you feel may be difficult. In time, AT can improve the way you react to stress, which is exactly what you want.

...AND RELAXING IN HALF AN HOUR

You have the techniques – now you can go even deeper, into a profoundly healing and revitalising state.

Lie comfortably as before, breathing diaphragmatically throughout, and go through the AT sequence at least once. Now, for the deeper stage, you have a choice: pictures or words.

Pictures

Some people are very good at visualising shapes and colours inside their heads. If you are one of these, then continue by seeing yourself lying on a warm, peaceful, sunlit beach. Imagine you are surrounded by a summer scene of blue sea, a paler sky with a few clouds and a long expanse of sand with perhaps a few trees round the edge.

You are lying warmed and protected by a beautiful light

which warms each part of your body in turn. Feel the light moving very slowly and peacefully from the neck down the spine, then up your arms from hand to shoulder and finally up your legs from foot to hip, releasing all your tensions and tightness as it goes. If your mind races – let it; make no effort to control your thoughts.

When you're ready, allow this picture to fade, and just lie in this profound state of peace until your time is up, when you clasp your hands together and get up very gently.

Words

If visualising is not your strong point, you can use verbal suggestions – a continuation, in fact, of the AT principle, but now at a still deeper level, encouraging psychological healing and emotional peace. These affirmations can be repeated silently as often as you wish; continue thereafter by simply resting in a deeply relaxed state.

You can make up your own, always positive, affirmations, or you can use the following ideas:

• Many of us lack confidence and this can make us irritable and exhausted. Repeat: 'I accept myself as I am. I use the power within me well.'
• For some of us, life is unfulfilling and frustrating; we seem to have taken the wrong turn. Repeat: 'I am finding the right life for me.'
• For others, the burden of what has happened in the past constantly drains us. Repeat: 'I let the past go, with love.'

As before, clasp your hands firmly when you get up, and take things very gently for a few moments until your energies are flowing again.

Whether you use pictures or words, you are very likely to fall asleep during this half-hour session. You may need a small bleeper to wake yourself up!

A *few words of explanation*

These imaging and verbal sequences are very powerful and, if practised over time, can cause helpful changes in your thoughts and emotions, aligning your energies in a more constructive and effective way. However, in this very deep state, memories and feelings that are usually kept hidden away may surface and swim up into your consciousness so that you can experience them, and eventually let them go. This happens to almost everyone and is part of a gradual, gentle healing process triggered by profound relaxation and the meditative state.

For more information

If you want to take this process further, consult your local library for information on meditation courses; or, for AT, send a stamped addressed envelope to the British Autogenic Society, c/o the Royal London Homeopathic Hospital, Great Ormond Street, London WC1 3HR.

FEEDING YOUR NERVES

A strong and resilient nervous system needs the right nourishment. When you are stressed the body tends to use up its nutrients more quickly and a shortage can stop you from coping well.

A good vitamin B complex and 500mg of vitamin C daily will help. But you need other nutrients, too (including soothing calcium) so make sure your diet at this challenging time is especially sound (liver and wheatgerm are outstanding stress-fighters).

For more on all these, see Chapter 4.

> *When you are stressed the body tends to use up its nutrients more quickly and a shortage can stop you from coping well*

COMPLEMENTARY MEDICINE
FOR YOUR NERVES

Medical herbalism

Consult a qualified practitioner for a prescription to soothe and strengthen your nervous system – better than a tranquilliser!

Homeopathy

Ask for Kali. Phos. biochemic tissue salt or a Kali. Phos. combination at your pharmacy or health food store; follow the stated dose. These excellent mineral salt remedies work within two to ten days to tone and refresh your nerves.

Ginseng helps you to deal with stress (see Chapter 4).

Reflexology and acupuncture

These are extremely relaxing therapies and, over time, can re-educate your nervous system; consult a qualified practitioner.

CHAPTER 9

Case History 4: James

J ames, aged 40, first sought treatment for tiredness about five years ago. His fatigue had built up over a period of time.

'I was teaching full-time then, with a lot of stress and problems. My immune system was under par, too, and I was picking up infections all the time. I would get an infection every six weeks or so, recover from it and then pick up another infection about six weeks after that.

'The lymph glands in my neck would often be swollen, and I had stiff muscles in the neck and shoulders, with irritation behind the eyes. I wasn't sleeping properly and I got very anxious about my health.'

James consulted his GP, who didn't know what was wrong with him.

'So I decided to have herbal treatment. I went to a herbal medicine clinic in Bristol where they were training practitioners, and they gave me a mixture of six herbs in a tincture. I took a standard dose of one teaspoonful in water three times a day.

'They gave me scullcap, a nerve tonic, borage to support the adrenal glands, clivers to cleanse the lymphatic system, echinacea to strengthen the immune system, heartsease to clear toxins from the body and wormwood for a tonic. The only other thing I took was vitamin C.

'It had been a long time before I sought treatment, so my recovery took time; it was about six months before I was completely better. Meantime, I developed an acute testicular condition so I urgently made an appointment to see a local herbalist, Laura Stannard. She then took over the whole treatment as it was easier for me to see someone locally than travelling to Bristol. She added Siberian ginseng (a general tonic and energiser) to my prescription, which was changed from time to time to take account of my improvement.'

James feels much better now and is much stronger. 'I don't get the fatigue I had before, I don't get infections all the time, my digestion is better; I still get stress but I am better able to cope with it. My testicular problem has cleared up, too. I no longer take the herbal medicine.

'I have been able to resume hill-walking, I swim and I play squash. (I have a degree, am studying for an MA, and work as a lecturer and as a consultant in education.)

'I was really happy with the treatment and would recommend anyone to see a herbalist for just about anything.'

CHAPTER 10

Depression and Fatigue

We all get depressed at some time or another. We feel tired, down, unwilling or unable to cope with life.

Some people feel low in winter when there is less natural daylight (see Energy from Nature: Light), and many women feel irritable and weepy before their periods (see Tired Body: Premenstrual Syndrome). Some women feel depressed after the birth of a baby, too. These low moods are temporary and they should pass off.

Life can deal terrible blows. Bereavement, loss, the suffering of someone you love, a long period of anxiety or illness, a crushing disappointment – as we try to deal with these heart-breaking experiences, depression is natural and understandable. This reactive depression is a necessary part of the long process of integration and healing.

Sadness that lingers longer than it should, however, is another matter. Depression that continues to eat into our lives, even when the reason for it is long gone – and perhaps when there seems to be no reason for it at all – is a major handicap and can be dangerous.

The causes for this kind of depression go deep. For instance, a lot of depression is not sadness at all, but suppressed anger; some people suffer from long-term depression because they cannot admit and express their rage and pain.

Deeper, more complex reasons for depression need skilled psychotherapy or psychiatric help. Really severe depression is a serious illness.

The questionnaire below will help you to identify the factors pointing to your depression.

ARE YOU DEPRESSED?

- Are you always tired, even after inactivity or rest?
- Does your daily life bore you most of the time, so that you take little interest in what is going on around you?
- Is everything an effort, something to be got through without energy or enthusiasm?
- Do you have a constant sense of failure?
- Are you burdened with feelings of guilt?
- Do you dislike yourself and believe you are unattractive?
- Do you think about death and suicide a lot?
- Do you cry often?
- Is decision-making difficult for you?
- Are you afraid of, and perhaps faced with, big changes in your life?
- Do you always expect the worst to happen?
- Do you get irritable very quickly over trivial things?
- Have you lost interest in sex?
- Have you lost your appetite lately, and are you losing weight?
- Have you noticed worrying health problems recently – for instance, painful or irregular periods, digestive upsets, candida (thrush), food allergies, insomnia, low blood sugar? (For the last three, see Tired Body.)
- Are you taking prescribed medication? (Some drugs cause depression; consult your GP.)
- Are you going through the menopause? (Consult a qualified nutritionist or a nutritionally informed doctor.)

If you answer Yes to seven or more of these questions, then you are likely to be depressed. The more Yeses that apply to you, the more depressed you are likely to be.

Note: The following advice is for people who feel they are mildly depressed, but who can still function reasonably well in their daily lives. Disabling depression needs skilled professional help; if you think this applies to you consult your doctor.

SELF-HELP FOR MILD DEPRESSION

USING NUTRITION

Deficiencies of B vitamins, in particular folic acid and B_{12}, are linked with depression. Take a strong vitamin B complex, together with 500mg of vitamin C, daily.

If you are on the Pill you may suffer from nutritional imbalances which can make your depression worse. As well as a vitamin B complex (which should contain B_6) and vitamin C, take the top recommended dose of zinc.

Foods to cut down or cut out are:
- caffeine (tea, coffee, chocolate, cola drinks)
- white sugar
- refined cereals and white flour foods
- junk foods
- alcohol

Eat regular meals; don't let yourself get ravenously hungry.

A lack of the Essential Fatty Acid **linolenic acid** is a factor in depression. Linolenic acid is plentiful in oily fish and there's even more in linseeds and linseed oil (these last two are available at your health food store).

The amino acid **phenylalanine** can relieve depression in a few days. Good food sources are:

- soybeans
- cottage cheese
- fish

- meat, especially poultry
- almonds, brazil nuts and pecans
- pumpkin and sesame seeds
- lima beans, chickpeas and lentils

See that these foods are generously supplied in your diet. If you wish to take phenylalanine as a supplement, consult a qualified naturopath or a nutritionally informed doctor.

> *St John's Wort is establishing a fine reputation for depression*

Hypericum, or **St John's Wort**, is establishing a fine reputation for depression. It is a highly effective remedy with few or no side effects. However, do not combine it with Prozac or any other tranquilliser, theophylline (bronchodilator), cyclosporin (immune suppressant), warfarin, digoxin, or the contraceptive pill. Take the recommended dose for at least four weeks to reap the full benefits.

GETTING YOURSELF OUT OF DEPRESSION

Do you know why you are depressed? Sit down with pen and paper and list the factors in your life – relationships, home life, health, money – that are making you depressed. Write down as well what makes you angry. Give yourself permission to be depressed for the time being.

This confrontation and clearing of your mind is the first step in helping yourself.

Helpful second steps
- Make up your mind to treat yourself as someone you appreciate and love.
- Decide to accept full responsibility for yourself and your life.
- Write down your strengths and talents.

- Work out what you want from life, both short- and long-term, and decide what changes you can make to get it; if there are factors you can't change, try to accept them without self-pity or rancour.
- Forgive yourself for making mistakes, past, present and future. The only person who never makes mistakes is someone who does absolutely nothing.
- Spoil yourself; choose a regular treat – even if it's only a weekly bunch of fresh flowers – and enjoy it.
- Decide on a creative activity you will enjoy, which is challenging and absorbing and which will bring you into contact with other people. You will be there to enjoy and not to win instant medals.
- A loving relationship is a strong bulwark against depression. How best can you cherish yours?
- Learn to relax: for how it's done, see the Stress and Fatigue chapter.
- Take some exercise and feel the instant benefits; see Energising Exercise.

Spoil yourself; choose a regular treat – and enjoy it

Because you may be anxious and confused, you may find clear thinking difficult and the idea of making changes very frightening. Is there a trusted friend you can talk all this through with?

COUNSELLING AND PSYCHOTHERAPY

Could psychotherapy or counselling help you? Sometimes, talking freely to someone who will understand and help you to see things more clearly (without telling you what to do) can help you recover.

The field of counselling and psychotherapy is growing rapidly and it must be said that not all practitioners are

> '*Depressed people are often trapped within their own personality but can release themselves, given the right help and guidance.*'
>
> Dr Andrew Stanway

competent and mature people. The best way to find skilled help is through recommendation.

In the absence of this, contact the addresses below.

For more information
Counselling: Send a 9″ × 6″ sae to the British Association for Counselling and Psychotherapy, Regent Place, Rugby, Warwickshire CV21 2PJ; telephone 01788 550899; website www.counselling.co.uk.

Psychotherapy: Send a 9″ × 6″ sae with two first-class stamps to the National Council of Psychotherapists, PO Box 6072, Nottingham NG6 9BW or telephone 0115 913 1382.

Complementary therapies
Acupuncture, reflexology, herbal and homeopathic medicine can all offer help against depression; consult your local library for a qualified practitioner.

CHAPTER 11

Energy from Nature

I n a natural world, your skin would be constantly exposed to water and sunlight, both exerting powerful effects on your energy and the way you feel. (Read Suzanne's case history, Chapter 12, for examples of nature cure at work.)

First, let's look at what water can do for your vitality and health.

WATER

Water treatments have been used since the time of Hippocrates in ancient Greece and continue today in European spas, clinics and hospitals. Modern hydrotherapy was pioneered by Sebastian Kneipp who was born in 1821, the son of a poor Bavarian weaver. The young Sebastian had TB and doctors told him he would soon die, but he read about water treatment and tried it on himself, eventually recovering completely. Later, as a priest, he gave water treatments to everyone – pope and peasant alike – who flocked to his home village, where flourishes today the largest spa centre in Europe.

Water on your skin can relax, rejuvenate, strengthen immunity and nerves, and help recovery from many illnesses. Here, we'll look at what it can do to ease stress and enhance well-being.

Very hot water exhausts you; warm water soothes

> *Water on your skin can relax, rejuvenate, strengthen immunity and nerves, and help recovery from many illnesses*

and relaxes; cold water speeds up your metabolism, stimulating the circulation and creating natural energy.

THE RELAXING BATH

Half-fill your bath with warm, not hot, water and add five drops each of essential oils of rosemary and geranium. While the water is running, take a loofah or a dry bath brush (preferably bristle) and brush your whole body, working upwards with firm strokes from feet to hips and along the arms from hands to shoulders. Brush your back and bottom with equal vigour, using gentler strokes for the stomach and leaving out face, neck and breasts. Dry skin brushing removes dead skin cells, stimulates circulation and promotes lymph drainage (the system that works with your bloodstream to remove impurities).

Get into your warm, fragrant bath and wash yourself all over with a flannel. You can relax for between ten and twenty minutes, topping up with warmer water from time to time.

Afterwards, use your favourite body lotion or make your own; add three drops of essential oil of rosemary, two drops of thyme and two drops of lavender to four ounces of carrier oil (cold-pressed jojoba, olive, almond or safflower are good.)

This bath is a marvellous relaxer for just before bedtime and will help you get a deep, refreshing night's sleep.

THE ENERGISING BATH

Use the same dry skin brushing and warm bath as before, but after you've washed yourself, run away some of the warm water and add cold so that the water quickly gets cooler. When it's as cold as you can comfortably stand, replace the plug and swish cool refreshing water all over your body. Get out and dry yourself vigorously with a rough towel.

By now your skin will be glowing and pink and you will feel marvellous; use body lotion to complete the session.

INSTANT ENERGY FROM WATER: THE SITZ BATH

If you need energy quickly and are fairly robust (see Warnings below), fill the bath at least halfway with cold water straight from the tap and immerse yourself so that the water comes up to your navel and your feet are resting on the end of the bath. Stay in this sitz bath for between thirty seconds and two minutes, then get out and rub yourself down briskly.

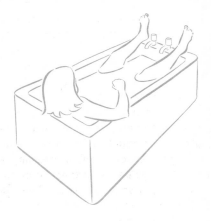

During a sitz bath, heartbeat slows and strengthens, circulation improves and the nervous system is stimulated. Cold water speeds up the elimination of wastes from lungs, bowels and bladder and, of course, skin; your skin throws off 500–900ml of sweat a day (particularly from glands in the armpits and groin) which can contain about 10g of wastes. (This process should not be suppressed, so go easy on the antiperspirants; a daily wash and a herbal deodorant should keep your armpits sweet and clean.)

Feet sitz

Just run cold water into a bucket or a bowl and rest your feet in it for a couple of minutes to refresh and revitalise yourself.

THE ENERGISING SHOWER

After a warm bath, run a cold shower, directing the jet all over your body and especially down your spine, for one minute; towel yourself vigorously afterwards.

Incidentally...

- Spraying cold water on the breasts will firm them and reduce congestion.
- Cold water sprayed on the face rejuvenates and firms the skin.
- A cold one-minute spray from foot to hip on each leg helps tone tired legs and minimise varicose veins.

> *Cold water sprayed on the face rejuvenates and firms the skin*

Used every day or so, water treatments can work wonders, relaxing and revitalising you and improving your general health.

WARNINGS

Don't use cold water treatments:

- after food
- when you are menstruating
- if you are very exhausted
- if you have high blood pressure, heart or respiratory disease
- if you suffer from thrombosis

Cold water should make you feel energetic, with your skin warm and glowing; if this doesn't happen, then you lack the vitality to respond and hydrotherapy is not right for you for the time being.

For more information
To find out more about hydrotherapy, consult a qualified naturopath.

LIGHT

We live, breathe and have our being in a sea of light. Nowadays, however, this is likely to be artificial much of the time; fluorescent and tungsten illuminate our world and, even when the sun goes down, we need never experience darkness.

However, our ability to replicate the light from the sun is only partial. Sunlight has qualities that most artificial lighting cannot match.

What's the difference between sunlight and ordinary artificial lighting, and does this difference have any effect on us?

THE POWER OF LIGHT

Natural light is a nutrient, like food. Its lack is most clearly seen during the winter months when, in spite of indoor lighting, many of us feel tired, lethargic and depressed – due to a lack of the right kind

> *Natural light is a nutrient, like food*

of light. This Seasonal Affective Disorder (SAD) grips its sufferers from December to March or April. Women are more susceptible than men, and SAD is most common in dark, foggy climates where natural light has trouble getting through.

For, although the lighting we use at home and at work is bright, it is incomplete compared with the full-spectrum light that comes from the sun. Natural daylight – which cannot pass in its entirety through ordinary window glass – has a direct effect upon the way our bodies work and how we feel.

Passing through the retina, natural light reaches the pineal gland in the forehead, called by the ancients the Third Eye and believed to be the seat of mysticism. There, it stops the release of a substance called melatonin. This hormone makes us sleepy and less alert and it slows us down, so it's not surprising that more melatonin is produced during the hours of darkness, tailing off at daybreak. Melatonin's effects are seasonal, as well; it influences our glandular system during the dark winter months, cutting down energy and sexual drive. When the spring sunshine arrives, melatonin levels decrease and we feel alert, bouncy and sexy again.

DO YOU GET SAD?

- Do you get depressed and tired during the winter months? Do you need more sleep then?
- Do you feel hungrier in the winter, craving starchy foods?
- Do you immediately start to feel better when the spring sunshine arrives?

If you answer Yes to these questions, then you may have SAD.

SELF-HELP FOR SAD

- Walk, or sit with eyes open or closed, in the sun for at least fifteen minutes daily, without spectacles or sunglasses. (NEVER look directly at the sun.)
- Daylight through windows, although incomplete, may help; try to work as close to a sunny window as possible.
- Mild SAD often responds to full-spectrum lighting or FSL (the nearest that technology can get to natural sunlight) which you can use at home; see the end of the chapter for details of a supplier.
- Consult your GP; some hospitals now offer FSL therapy for severe SAD.

THE BENEFITS OF NATURAL LIGHT

In spite of justified warnings on the dangers of too much bright sunlight, moderate natural light is absolutely vital for good health.

Light researcher Dr Damien Downing has found that we are short-changing ourselves on the benefits of natural light. We all know that a walk in the sun makes us feel better, more energetic and optimistic, but there's much more to it than that; we actually need natural light.

Under fluorescent light, people can get irritable and tired, with impaired vision; laboratory rabbits will even eat their young and some fruits refuse to ripen.

Sunlight enters your body in two ways; not only via the eyes, but also through the skin, where it causes vitamin D to be made and absorbed into the body to facilitate the use of calcium and magnesium.

Moderate natural light is absolutely vital for good health

Natural daylight:
- strengthens our immune system and bones
- speeds recovery from many illnesses, including ME
- helps wounds and sores to heal
- improves eczema and psoriasis

When our skin is exposed to natural light:
- the bloodstream is irradiated
- the oxygen-carrying capacity of the blood goes up by as much as 50 per cent, leaving the heart and lungs with less work to do
- excess cholesterol and high blood pressure tend to go down
- muscles increase their strength and staying power

So – how can we enjoy the benefits of light without getting burned to a crisp, or worse?

SAFE SUN

How long you should stay in the sun depends on two factors:
- how brightly it is shining
- your skin type

The sun is at its hottest at midday during June, July and August (it probably isn't possible to tan at all under a weak January sun). The paler your skin, the shorter should be your exposure.

Find out how long you can stay in bright, hot summer sunshine without discomfort, and halve it. This is your MED (Minimal Erythema Dose). In hot sun you can increase your MED time by about one minute per day, but go carefully.

Use a good sunscreen, but remember that staying in the sun too long, even with a sunscreen, can be dangerous, so stick to your MED with or without sunblock.

In fact, even if you enjoy the sunshine in loose, covering clothes and a straw hat (but without specs or sunglasses), you can still reap many benefits that way.

For more information
Full spectrum lighting: Contact FSL at 19 Lincoln Road, Cressex Business Park, High Wycombe, Bucks HP12 3FX; telephone 014945 26051.
SAD: Send an sae to the SAD Association at PO Box 989, Steyning, West Sussex BN44 3HG; telephone 01903 814942.

CHAPTER 12

Case History 5: Suzanne

N aturopathy, or nature cure, uses natural foods, exercise, relaxation, water and sunlight to trigger the body into detoxifying and healing itself.

Suzanne, aged twenty, is a student at the British College of Naturopathy and Osteopathy in North London.

'In about April 1997 I began to notice that I was tiring very quickly. I was studying full-time and – I've always been very active – I would swim nearly every day and visit the gym regularly, but this gradually became impossible. By September I was sleeping twelve hours a day and coughing a lot at night.

'In the end I couldn't go to college full-time any more, and it was suggested I might have ME. I went to hospital and they did several tests – although not for ME – and found everything was normal except for one enzyme in the liver which was very active. This could have been a sign that I was recovering from a viral illness.'

Suzanne didn't want to take any drugs, so she consulted a lecturer at her college.

'I had to keep a diet diary over seven days, putting down everything I ate and drank. He put me on a strict diet. First thing in the morning I had lemon juice, freshly squeezed, and chopped apple for breakfast.

'Throughout the day I had to eat every two or three hours to stop myself getting really tired. I would nibble sesame seeds, sunflower seeds, almonds, dried apricots, pineapple, papaya. I had to cut out wheat, pasta and hard cheeses; I had never drunk cow's milk anyway so giving it up wasn't a problem. Lunch was based on rice with live yogurt, sometimes eggs or fish, vegetables. In the afternoon I would have grapes, blackcurrants. I had no tea or coffee and no white sugar. At teatime

I would have some nettle tea. Supper would be rice-based again, with fish, especially mackerel and fresh salmon.

'For six weeks I also took supplements, including kelp tablets and brewer's yeast.'

As well as a diet which cleanses the body, naturopathy uses water. 'I took a short cold bath every morning, and I used hot and cold compresses on my neck which brought down my swollen glands.

'I had to do lots of breathing, from the stomach. I had been breathing with my upper chest, and the lower ribs and diaphragm were not working at all. My upper spine was restricted and my neck very tight; they gave me osteopathy for this and some stretching exercises.

'I completed my naturopathic treatment with short walks in the sunshine every day.'

Suzanne had to keep going for four or five weeks before she noticed any improvement. 'When I started to feel better I did a couple of fasts. After that I felt marvellous; my brain was so clear and I had so much energy.'

It took about ten months for Suzanne to recover completely. 'I think that my fatigue was linked to babyhood meningitis and later glandular fever which I had as a teenager; my practitioner thought so, too. I haven't had any infections or illnesses since and my energy is very good; I am swimming and working out again in the gym. I have a good diet now, but it is less strict.

'I am very pleased to be training for a profession that is so helpful; I am living proof of its effectiveness.'

CHAPTER 13

Body Clocks: the Science of Rhythm

F or every living creature on the planet, time moves in cycles – winter to spring, dark into light, low tide and high tide. In obedience to these natural rhythms, we have internal body clocks which influence every moment of our lives.

> 'To every thing there is a season, and a time to every purpose under the heaven'
>
> Ecclesiastes 3:1

Do you feel lethargic in the winter months? Your annual body clock responds each autumn to shorter, darker days by slowing you down.

Do you suffer from premenstrual miseries? Your monthly clock triggers body changes in the days before your period begins.

The science of biological rhythms (chronobiology) is fast discovering ways in which many natural cycles – daily, monthly and yearly – hold sway over our energies, our moods, our thinking, our sexual drive and our susceptibility to illness. Inside our bodies, there are daily fluctuations in our temperature, brain waves, blood pressure, heartbeat, hormonal output, digestion and even the division of body cells. It's no wonder we notice swings in our moods and, in our energy, peaks and troughs.

(Chronobiology is not to be confused with 'biorhythms', which are based on the idea that cyclical changes can be worked out mathematically using,

> Many natural cycles hold sway over our energies, our moods, our thinking, our sexual drive and our susceptibility to illness

as a starting point, astrological signs.)

With an understanding of biological rhythms, it's now possible to work *with* these powerful forces, instead of against them. Indeed, one of the secrets of boundless energy and youthfulness may lie in listening to what these rhythms – both in the natural world and inside ourselves – have to tell us.

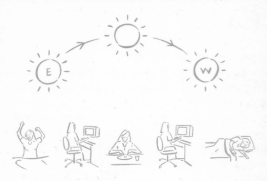

Biological rhythms originated as a response to the sun and we still obey sunrise and sunset. Volunteers living in underground caves with no natural light or any other time cues still obey sleeping and waking cycles based on the sun.

Some people – especially women, and those who live alone – have slightly shorter daily cycles, but these small variations are constantly being corrected in our every day lives; major controlling factors are regular mealtimes, the working day and, of course, our meters of man-made time, watches and clocks.

STOPPING THE CLOCK

What happens if these rhythms are thrown into confusion? The most dramatic example is jet lag. After a journey across time zones we can feel terrible, both physically and mentally. Tests carried out by the United States Army found that soldiers flown to Europe took several days to recover their ability to think clearly.

Shift workers on duty all night one week and all day the next often suffer from fatigue and irritability as their bodies try to adjust to this muddled schedule.

But getting your rhythms out of synch is not only unpleasant – it can also damage your health. Airline pilots, who frequently travel across time zones, tend to suffer from fatigue, digestive problems, headaches, cramps, insomnia and emotional problems more than other people.

Body clocks are vulnerable, too. Stress can disrupt your natural cycles with the release of hormones that constantly kick you into a state of alarm. Biological rhythms tend to get shorter with age, and their flexibility varies from one person to another.

Understanding natural rhythms helps us to take advantage of them, for better health and increased vitality.

> *Understanding natural rhythms helps us to take advantage of them*

THE NINETY-MINUTE CYCLE

Your ability to concentrate lasts about ninety minutes at one time, after which you tend to daydream. (If you're tired or stressed, this time will be shorter.) So, to get the most out of yourself with the least effort, break off work for a short while after ninety minutes and come back to it later.

Energy fluctuates at the same rate. Every ninety minutes, you may feel tired and lethargic for a few moments; this will soon pass. If you are driving long distances, a short break to take account of this drop is a sensible idea.

You may also feel slightly peckish every ninety minutes or so. You're probably not truly hungry, only at the mercy of your own body clock, and this urge will soon wear off; a glass of mineral water is a good substitute for something fattening!

You may also need to urinate every ninety minutes or, if you're a smoker, you may want a cigarette. (If you're trying to cut down, a useful tip is to take plenty of deep breaths and promise yourself a puff the next time around.)

DAILY CYCLES

Are you a lark or an owl?
- Do you wake up early and go to bed early?
- Do you usually get up feeling full of energy and raring to go?
- Do you work best in the mornings?

If you answer Yes to these questions, this means you are a lark.

- Do you wake up late and go to bed late?
- Do you crawl out of bed feeling sluggish, struggle through the morning, and feel most alive in the evening, when you're ready for anything?

If you answer Yes to these questions, this makes you an owl.

It's much easier to cope if you know what type you are and plan your days accordingly. (Let's hope you don't marry your opposite…)

BODY CLOCK EATING

If you're dieting, it's helpful to know that, because digestive hormones have different tasks for different times in the day, calories eaten early in the day are more likely to be burned off in activity than calories eaten later, which are laid down as fat; this natural cycle is designed to give us energy when we need it.

SLEEP RHYTHMS

Sleep itself goes in cycles, from light sleep to the deep sleep periods during which you dream. Sleep stimulates growth and healing, restores body and mind, sorts out your daily experiences for you, enables you to learn and above all gives you energy for the next day.

If you have trouble sleeping, see Tired Body, Insomnia, for advice.

THE SIESTA AND POWER-NAPPING

The lowest energy point in the twenty-four cycle, apart from between 3 and 5 a.m. when we're asleep, is just after lunch (especially true if you've had pasta and alcohol, and if you're a lark).

Nature probably intended us to take a nap in the early afternoon because in many climates it is the hottest time of day; this tradition still continues in sunny countries, when all activities cease for the siesta.

Many high-flyers swear by short 'power-naps' which rest and revitalise. Churchill, a workaholic and regular power-napper, wrote: 'Nature had not intended man to work from eight in the morning until midnight without the refreshment of blessed oblivion, which, even if it lasts only twenty minutes, is sufficient to renew all vital forces.'

About half of college students nap regularly. Those taking a nap before a big exam were found to do better (but try it out first – beginners can feel awful when they get up!)

The best length is about twenty minutes; if you nap too long you may find it hard to sleep that night. The best time is just after lunch. If you can, find a quiet room with a

A walk in the open air will refresh you and get you past that after-lunch slump

comfortable chair and use a timer. Even office workers can put their feet up for a while in the quiet lunchtime. For how to relax completely, see the Stress and Fatigue chapter.

If napping is not for you, a walk in the open air will refresh you and get you past that after-lunch slump.

MOON MOODS

Our nearest heavenly body, the moon exerts a tremendous pull as she circles the earth, causing tides to rise and fall and even the earth's crust to bulge and recede by several inches. Primitive peoples believed that the moon had mystical powers and that the full moon could drive you mad.

A woman's menstrual cycle is based on the moon's phases, although it does not always follow this monthly rhythm exactly. Premenstrual hormonal changes can inflict fatigue, depression and irritability, as well as fluid retention and aches and pains. (Apparently, men have lunar cycles too; they can suffer from mood swings and weight gains as well.) If you are plagued with Premenstrual Syndrome, listen to your body. Try to take more rest and avoid stress until hormonal adjustments allow you to feel confident and energetic again.

For more advice on PMS, see Tired Body, Premenstrual Syndrome.

YEARLY CYCLES

In the winter months when there is less daylight some people suffer from fatigue and depression. This Seasonal Affective Disorder (SAD) is caused by changes in production of the light-sensitive hormone melatonin. The best way round this is to get as much natural light as you can during the winter months; a fifteen-minute walk in daylight every day can lift low spirits. Full-spectrum lighting at home may help.

For more advice on SAD, see Energy from Nature, Light.

Natural light has profound and widespread effects on our physical and emotional health and, when the summer sun arrives, we notice a lightening of mood and greater energy. Natural sunlight is a vital part of the annual cycle for all living things.

LIFESTYLE RHYTHMS

The natural world follows its own rhythms. But the human animal, with his increasingly artificial environment, often forgets these ancient cycles which are so neces-

After exertion and challenge, we need to unwind

sary for our well-being. Perhaps this is why we tend to neglect the highs and lows of our individual lives.

In the same way that spring and summer's activities are followed by winter's quiet, our body rhythms demand that, after exertion and challenge, we need to unwind, to balance the equation with a compensating downturn of energy. Few of us plan for this recovery time, but to do so makes sure that we have the extra energy and resources the next time they are needed. Even the most level and repetitive lifestyle has peaks and troughs which we need to recognise and accept.

So – leave gaps between stressful times if you can. Remember that major changes in your life – getting married, moving house, changing your job, having a baby, dealing with family loss – can distort your body rhythms and drain your energies. Make allowances for these heavy demands.

In the way that you live your life, try to co-operate with both your own body clocks and the rhythms of the natural world around you, with which your existence is inextricably linked.

CHAPTER 14

Energising Exercise

*S*urely, if we are tired, exercise will simply make us feel worse? What's the point in forcing an already tired body to move, when all it wants to do is rest?

To some extent, of course, this is common sense and true. If you are absolutely exhausted or ill (particularly if you have ME) and you indulge in a bout of strenuous exercise, this is just not sensible.

But if you are one of those people who feel lethargic and under par much of the time, exercise could be just what you need to give you stamina and vitality.

Here are the reasons why.

When we are stressed – common nowadays! – our bodies produce a lot of adrenalin to help us deal with the problems we are facing. After the crisis is over, any adrenalin left in the system is dispersed through natural movement.

However, our modern way of living often excludes vigorous activity, so this adrenalin build-up remains, decreasing the efficiency of the heart, affecting the brain and making us irritable and tired. Not only that – inactivity makes muscles tense and stiff, so that we feel less inclined to exercise than ever.

Lack of exercise, therefore, puts us into a downward spiral which affects both well-being and mood, turning us into tired, fed-up couch potatoes.

GET STARTED!

'Movement is strong medicine,' says Herbert de Vries, researcher at the University of Southern California, where a team of scientists found that a single bout of exercise works

> *Exercise works better than a tranquilliser against stiff muscles, anxiety and tension*

better than a tranquilliser against stiff muscles, anxiety and tension.

Exercise gives you more energy. With regular exercise, there is an increase in the energy-producing power of body cells so that energy is released, not only more quickly, but in larger amounts.

Exercise sparks you into more activity. Says Dr Lawrence Lamb, cardiologist and fitness consultant, 'Exercise will get the metabolic machinery out of inertia, and you'll be refreshed and ready to go.'

So, when you turn up at your dance class, or the local tennis court, saying to yourself, 'I can't possibly do this; I want to go home and put my feet up,' stay and give it a try. Unless you are truly depleted or ill, you will find that after a while your favourite exercise lifts your mood and causes your energies to come flooding back.

EXERCISE AND DEPRESSION

Exercise is better than an antidepressant – and without the side effects. Some doctors now recommend it as part of their treatment regime against depression.

University students who complained of feeling depressed were divided into two groups; one group received psychotherapy and the other went running every day. After ten weeks the runners had overtaken the others; they felt better, worked harder and did better in their exams.

How does this happen?

Our bodies produce natural mood-enhancing chemicals, making us feel cheerful, confident and

> *Exercise is better than an antidepressant – and without the side effects*

energetic. With strenuous exercise, levels of these chemicals shoot up to such an extent – by about 145 per cent – that some exercisers can get addicted to their sport. And that's not all – because of brain changes during strenuous exercise, enthusiasts report entering into a calm, meditative mood, a state of bliss. It's not surprising that many people feel they can't live without their euphoric high.

Let's not forget what exercise does for our physical health, too:

- strengthens heart and lungs
- cuts the risk of heart disease and stroke
- improves circulation
- strengthens muscles
- keeps tendons flexible and joints mobile
- increases the blood supply to the brain so we can think more clearly
- increases the body's metabolic rate so that we use up our calories faster instead of accumulating them as fat

When you think about it, all this isn't surprising. After all, our bodies were made to exercise – to run, swim, climb, dance, make love. Summarising the scientific view of its benefits, leading health author Leslie Kenton writes in *The Joy of Beauty* (Century Arrow): 'Some even believe that this is because regular strenuous movement is a natural need of human beings, one for which we have been genetically programmed and one which, if denied over a period of time, leads to feelings of timidity, negativity, lack of creativity, and chronic fatigue as well as physical illness.'

WHAT KIND OF EXERCISE?

Outdoors
Outdoor sports – tennis, swimming, cycling, running – are easy to find. There are health clubs and sports centres

in most neighbourhoods; consult your local library for information. As well as the companionship and fun that most exercise offers, outdoor exercise adds the extra benefits of natural light (see Energy from Nature, Light).

Walking   Never underestimate the health benefits of walking, which seems so peaceful and undemanding. If you walk regularly in the open air, you will:

- strengthen heart and lungs
- help to keep your cholesterol levels healthy
- improve your general fitness

> *Never underestimate the health benefits of walking*

Enjoy gentle walking with congenial companions in beautiful surroundings, and you will find you have all the energy you need for the miles you will cover (although it's not a good idea to start off with a marathon hike!).

Your walking can range from taking the dog round the park to rambling days and walking holidays. If you are doing some serious walking, make sure you have the right clothes – particularly a good stout pair of boots.

Indoors

Indoor sports and exercise classes – martial arts, badminton, indoor swimming, aerobics and dance classes – are plentiful; again, visit your local library, or evening institute, for more information.

Sports generally develop speed, strength, stamina and concentration. If you choose a fitness – or, better still, a dance – class, you can add to the above qualities suppleness, rhythm and co-ordination.

Dance is a huge field, from ballroom dancing to jazz and modern dance. (Ballet is a marvellous system of physical training but if you come to it as an adult you may find some of the exercises difficult.) Jazz dance is especially good, with its strong emphasis on a lithe body and a flexible spine, and because it is done to music with a strong beat and is so expressive, it can energise you and lift your spirits in a very short time.

Any exercise that makes your heart and lungs work harder is **aerobic**. **Anaerobic** exercise (for example, weight-lifting) is done for a shorter time and concentrates on strengthening the muscles.

STARTING TO EXERCISE

To begin with, pace yourself. Start slowly, increasing your exercise time and level of difficulty as you get fitter; remember that the only person you are competing with is yourself. It's a good idea to exercise one day and leave out the next, giving your body a chance to recover and adjust.

> *It's a good idea to exercise one day and leave out the next*

Check with your doctor first if you suffer from:
- chest pains
- leg pains when walking
- swollen ankles
- shortness of breath after mild exercise

Choose a form of exercise, above all, that you enjoy. Can you afford it? Will it fit into your lifestyle without strain and stress? If it won't, then you're not very likely to keep it up – and persistence is the only way to reap the benefits.

Guidelines
- Never exercise after a heavy meal. Wait, preferably for two hours, before starting.

- If your stomach is empty, have just a small snack (a cup of milk and a biscuit will do) to give you the fuel you need.
- Never exercise if you are totally exhausted or ill.
- Never exercise to the point where you are so out of breath you can't even talk.
- Always make sure you have suitable and comfortable clothes which will keep you warm enough and which you can shed in layers if necessary.
- After your exercise, take a few moments to cool down and relax; drink a glass of water to replace the fluids you have lost.

WARMING UP

If you're out of practice, or just need to warm up before an exercise session, here are some easy movements to stretch and tone your body and get you started.

Wear comfortable clothes and find a suitable place to work in. Throughout these exercises, which should be done gently and slowly, don't forget to breathe!

1. Upward stretch
Stand, feet a little apart, and stretch up, trying to touch the ceiling (let your shoulders relax); breathe in. Relax down, bending your knees and allowing your hands to brush the floor; breathe out. Repeat up to ten times.

2. Side stretch
Standing upright, feet a little apart, stretch your arms out to the sides. Keeping them there, turn your upper body to one side, twisting at the waist and keeping the hips still, then to the other. Repeat up to ten times in each direction.

3. Hip circles
Stand, with hands on hips, and rotate your hips in a big circle, first in one direction and then in the other, twisting at

the waist. Repeat up to ten times in each direction.

4. Cycling
Lie on the floor on your back, and lift your bent legs. Pedal slowly in the air for up to one minute.

5. Stomach lift
If you haven't got time for the other warm-ups, at least do this one! This wonderful stomach lift is essential for a flat, firm stomach and youthful appearance, and it massages the internal organs as well.

Stand feet apart, knees slightly bent, hands on knees. Pull your stomach in and up very slightly, and hold the contraction; without relaxing, pull in again a little further, and again hold; finally, pull your stomach in and up as far as you can and hold it there for a count of ten (this final pull is easier if you hold your breath). Relax. Repeat at least three times.

OTHER PATHWAYS TO ENERGY
THE ALEXANDER TECHNIQUE

F. Matthias Alexander, an Australian actor born in 1869, developed voice loss which threatened his career.

However, instead of just giving up, he spent many years studying the habits of posture and body use which can cause vocal and many other health problems. Having recovered the use of his voice, he taught his technique of better body use in both England and America for many years, and the Alexander Method is widely used and taught today.

Alexander lessons, which are given one-to-one, aim to re-educate our habitual, and often faulty, ways of moving and holding ourselves. The teacher makes the pupil aware of what he or she is doing, and how body use is interfering with health. A light corrective touch is often all that is needed to guide the pupil into a sense of lengthening and expanding his or her body, with a feeling of freedom, lightness and easier movement.

The Alexander Technique can relieve all kinds of disorders, particularly stress-related back and neck problems, poor breathing, and fatigue.

For more information
Contact The Society of Teachers of Alexander Technique, 129 Camden Mews, London NW1 9AH; telephone 020 7284 3338; website www.stat.org.uk.

YOGA

The East has taught us much in recent years and the popularity of yoga is part of this trend. In yoga – meaning 'yoke' – body, mind and spirit cannot be separated. Yoga has a profound effect, not only on your energy, suppleness and fitness, but upon all body systems including the glands and nerves, and upon your psychological and emotional well-being, too.

> *Yoga has a profound effect on all body systems*

Yoga exercises vary, but broadly they are a series of slow, calm poses, usually involving stretching and breathing. They encourage a healthy, harmonious body and a tranquil mind. Advanced yoga includes deep meditation and offers a whole philosophy of living.

'Real, sustainable inner peace involves no effort and engenders no fatigue,' writes Dr Robin Monro in his book *Yoga for Common Ailments* (for full details see page 17). 'Yoga is a way of living – a means of achieving health in body, mind and spirit. For it to be effective, however, you must make it a part of your life and practise daily.'

For what yoga can do to combat fatigue, see Jason's case history on page 19.

For more information

Contact your local library for information on local classes. There are many branches of yoga; hatha yoga is the most commonly used in the West.

CHI KUNG

The arts of energy practised by the ancients are now known by the Chinese name of Chi Kung (another name for Qigong). 'Chi' means energy and 'Kung' means art.

This ancient system was revived in modern China and is now becoming better known and appreciated in the West.

Like yoga, its deceptively gentle movements and breathing exercises can be used to improve your health and energy, or it can be taken much further. As Wong Kiew Kit writes in his recent book *Chi Kung for Health and Vitality* (Element Books), Chi Kung refers to the 'art of developing life energy for health, internal power, mind cultivation and spiritual fulfilment'. Like yoga, Chi Kung needs care and patience to yield its full benefits.

I describe here one of the foremost Chi Kung exercises, to whet your appetite for this harmonising and energising system. My source is Wong Kiew Kit's book.

Lifting the sky

Stand with your feet fairly close together and your arms hanging down at your sides. Pause for a few seconds to feel yourself relax. Then smile, from the heart – don't worry, you won't look silly – and allow your smile to lift your spirits.

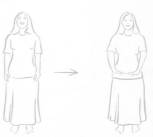

Next, place your straight arms down in front of you, elbows turned outwards, and lift your hands so that they are at right angles to your arms, with wrists arched and fingers almost meeting in front of your body.

Holding this position with straight arms, slowly stretch your arms a little downwards and then forwards and upwards in a continuous arc, at the same time breathing in very gently through your nose. As you perform this sweeping arc, imagine energy flowing into you.

When your arms are right above your head, pause a moment, and then push your arms upwards as high as you can, as though you are trying to lift the sky.

Lastly, lower your arms to your sides, arms straight and hands stretched out in the same line, like a bird flapping its wings. At the same time, breathe out gently through the mouth. As you breathe out, imagine negative, destructive energy being drained away.

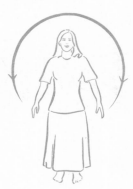

You can repeat this marvellous exercise up to thirty times.

For more information
For information on classes nationwide, contact: Wu's Tai Chi Chuan Academy (London UK), 34 Osnaburgh Street, London NW1 2ND; telephone 020 7916 6064; website www.wustyle-europe.com.

CHAPTER 15

Energy and Your Job

By Friday, do you feel headachy and tired, with perhaps poor concentration, a runny nose, itchy skin and even nausea? If all this wears off over the weekend and starts again during your working week you could be one of the many victims of Sick Building Syndrome. SBS is an umbrella term describing the malaise of those who work in offices, hospitals, or even private houses, and which is actually caused by the working environment itself.

> If you hate your job, it could be your workplace that's causing the trouble

Recognised by the World Health Organisation, SBS affects more women than men (perhaps because women spend more time actually in the office in front of a VDU), and occurs more often in new or recently refurbished office buildings. So, if you hate your job, it could be your workplace that's causing the trouble.

How can a place of work sap your energy and upset your health?

CONCRETE JUNGLE

The modern office block is an unnatural environment. Light is mostly artificial, air stale and recycled, and office equipment and new furnishings a source of chemical fumes. The atmosphere may be too dry or too damp and temperatures too hot or too cold. These environmental stressors can, at the least, make you feel listless and under par, and at the worst actually make you ill.

Glare from fluorescent lighting, shiny walls, glass-covered tables or large windows exposed to hot sunlight can cause eyestrain, headaches and fatigue.

In addition, **fluorescent lighting** offers an incomplete light spectrum (more distorted than tungsten) which can make clear vision difficult. The healthy full spectrum of natural daylight is partly blocked by ordinary window glass.

Air-conditioning plants can be badly designed or poorly maintained, simply shunting stale air endlessly from one office to another and providing an ideal transport system for bacteria, viruses and pollutants. About 75 per cent of the smoke from a cigarette goes into the air, to be circulated and breathed in by everybody else.

Harmful bacteria thrive in high humidity, whereas a very dry atmosphere can cause dry throat, nose and eyes with dry, itchy skin.

Some heating systems are set too high, making concentration difficult and causing fatigue and discomfort, and in most new office buildings you can't even open the windows to let in fresh air.

High-voltage metal drums and carbon-based toners in **modern copiers** give off toxic chemical vapours and their chemically coated paper can cause skin irritation.

It's no mystery that SBS is most common in **recently furnished offices** – the chemical fumes initially given off by newly installed synthetic carpets, upholstery and plywood add their pollutants to the atmosphere. Your friendly cleaning lady may use **sprays** giving off unpleasant fumes which linger around just when you arrive in the morning.

Open plan offices are sometimes designed in such a way that no one gets any privacy and people feel they have no control over their own working space. The recent 'hot-desking' vogue means that people park their laptops wherever there's a free desk so they have no permanent workstation, either, and this doesn't suit everybody. **Noise** from adjacent copiers, printers, phones and so on makes an already stressful environment even worse.

VDUS

The Extremely Low Frequency (ELF) radiation given off by VDUs is generally lower than it used to be, and various screens are available which offer some protection. However, scientists continue to study the probable links between ELF and problems with health (the jury is still out on possible risks to pregnant women from VDUs). Over time, VDUs can cause deterioration in focusing with headaches and fatigue (made worse by a flickering screen), and long hours without a break can encourage eye muscles to spasm.

Poor seating and posture, with overuse, increase the risk of wrist damage (Repetitive Strain Injury).

MOBILE PHONES

Do you use a mobile phone to carry your office around with you? Swedish researchers found that mobile phone users reported headaches, fatigue, and 'hot face'. The low-level radiation given off may be why prolonged use – about thirty-five minutes – can cause a small rise in blood pressure. Headsets do not always give protection and may even increase levels of radiation.

So – play safe and keep your calls short.

SURVIVING

How much say do you have in the way your office is run? Ask your employers to make sure that:

- air-conditioning filters are regularly cleaned
- copiers and printers are kept well away from main working spaces
- carbonless copy paper is not stored on open shelves

Sound can be absorbed by carpets, acoustic partitions, padded sight screens and soft furnishings.

Tests have found that **full-spectrum lighting** promotes better vision (see the end of the chapter for supplier). A **desk lamp** will give you control over your own lighting space.

People with **open windows** or **desk fans** are sick less often; a small desk fan will move stale air around and give a refreshing and revitalising cool breeze.

> *A small desk fan will move stale air around and give a refreshing and revitalising cool breeze*

Negative ions – electrical particles created by sunlight and thunderstorms and plentiful near plants and running water – are a natural way of mopping up air pollution. Companies that have installed negative ionisers in their offices report less illness and better-tempered and more alert employees.

Positive ions, which can make people irritable and tired, are increased by:

- fluorescent lighting
- air conditioning
- cigarette smoke
- modern electronic office equipment

A small portable ioniser could improve your well-being at work, particularly if you suffer from hay fever (see the end of the chapter for supplier).

A simple way of **improving your working space** is to put a bowl of fresh water on your desk containing a few drops of essential oil of lemon grass, lemon, pine or thyme. Or treat yourself to a plant; a NASA study found that almost every plant they tested diffused office chemicals and added moisture and oxygen to the air. A bowl of growing chrysanthemums clears the surrounding air in about six weeks.

To cut **VDU** static:
- grow a cactus *Cerus Peruvianus*, on your desk
- sprinkle water on the carpet
- wear leather-soled shoes
- use anti-stat screens and mats

If your **skin is dry**, spray your face and refresh yourself with mineral water or rosewater from a plastic bottle. For a quick pick-me-up, drink mineral or filtered water with ice from the office fridge.

New keyboards minimise **wrist fatigue** and the danger of RSI; check your posture and seating, and take a ten-minute break from your VDU every hour if you can.

For **tired eyes**, close them and cover them with cupped palms, without pressure; stay like this for a few moments to give your eyes a welcome rest. Or use acupressure to improve your sight; press firmly on the inside corners of both eyes with middle fingers for several seconds, release and press again. Repeat as often as you like. To give eye muscles a rest from focusing on the screen break off from your VDU occasionally to gaze into the distance for a few moments.

Lastly, try to get a **walk outside**, preferably in the nearest park, in the lunch hour and on the way to and from work every day for fresh air and natural light.

For more information
For more about office health: Call the Health and Safety

Executive Helpline on 0541 545500 or write to HSE Information Centre, Broad Lane, Sheffield S3 7HQ; alternatively contact your local environmental health officer.

For full-spectrum lighting: Contact FSL at 19 Lincoln Road, Cressex Business Park, High Wycombe, Bucks HP12 3FX; telephone 014945 26051.

For ionisers: Contact the Wholistic Research Company at The Old Forge, Mill Green, Hatfield, Hertfordshire AL9 5NZ; telephone 01707 262686; fax 01707 258828; website www.wholisticresearch.com.

CHAPTER 16

Work Addiction

Are you one of those people who just can't stop working? Do you flog yourself to get absolutely everything done at work, every time, no matter how tired you are? Are you a workaholic?

Work addiction is a modern health hazard. Once, its victims were mostly men but today's women, trying to satisfy the demands of both job and home, or just making their way in what can still be a male-dominated workplace, are equally vulnerable.

Some women at home are workaholics, too. They feel they must hand-knit the children's sweaters, make their own

> *Work addiction is a modern health hazard*

biscuits and ice-cream, paint the house unaided and then fit in an aerobics class afterwards, getting back just in time to slump, exhausted, at the table while the family tucks into their lovely home-made bread. (Divorced women apparently do better in business than their married sisters; do they feel the need to prove themselves after a broken relationship, or do they simply have more time to devote to work?)

In these days of electronic communication, more and more people are working from home and this, paradoxically, can lead to overwork. Used to a structured office routine, some people can't pace themselves and neglect to stop for trivialities like meals and bed.

Some self-employed workers feel guilty about stopping for a break. Because the work often comes in fits and starts, it's hard to set limits and feel confident that more work will turn up when you are ready for it.

And many of us get caught in a spiral of costs as we spend more and more money (which has to be earned) in an attempt to keep up with the materialistic, money-obsessed world we live in.

Whatever the reason for it, work addiction carries a health warning. With continuous long-term overwork, fatigue interferes with clear thinking and work output goes, not up as we hope, but down.

By creating their own stresses, workaholics force their bodies to produce stress-fighting hormones more and more often, giving them an adrenalin high. When this mechanism becomes so exhausted that it can't respond any more, severe fatigue sets in, which can even lead to ME (for more about ME see Tired Body).

Dr Peter Nixon, heart expert, warns, 'We go over the top into exhaustion and deteriorating function if we allow ourselves to be aroused to make effort and struggle beyond the level of healthy fatigue.'

However, there's another side to this. Some people work all hours and love it. A creative attitude to work, so that you see it as a game, a challenge, a wonderful country to be explored, fires you with enthusiasm and zest and will overcome obstacles and disasters. These lucky people have to be prised away from their beloved work by friends and family so they can enjoy the other blessings in life…

ARE YOU A WORKAHOLIC?

- Do you take little interest in anything outside your job?
- Do you feel guilty and at a loose end on holiday?
- Do you find it difficult or impossible to hand your work over to someone else for the time being?
- Do you use your work to fill gaps in your life – loneliness, lack of interesting activities, an inability to relate to other people?

- Do you find it hard to accept criticism about your work, while having a huge need for praise?
- Do you find it hard to forgive yourself for making mistakes at work?
- Do you like everyone to think you are indispensable in your job?
- When socialising, do you find it important to mention your work, feeling that it defines, totally, what you are?
- Do you feel better with a rigidly planned life?
- Do you take on so many things that you can't concentrate on, or finish satisfactorily, one thing?
- Do you resent the way you have to work?

If you answer Yes to most of these questions you are probably addicted to your work.

Fatigue will be part of your lifestyle; you're so used to it that you don't notice it any more. Relaxing, letting go of your work responsibilities, thinking about something else – you regard all this as a waste of time and not on your agenda.

What is meant by 'work addiction'?
Addiction to anything means you can't do without it; the word comes from the Latin, *addicere*, to surrender.

Obviously, it's better to be addicted to your job than to heroin or cocaine, but the principle is the same. The substance or activity to which you are addicted is vitally necessary to you and fills a gap in your life. It is controlling you – you are not controlling it.

GIVING UP WORK ADDICTION

Letting go of any addiction takes time, effort and courage – but it's worth it.

Start by limiting the hours you give to your job, filling the gap you create with something that will bring quick rewards in terms of pleasure. Find other areas in your life where you can grow, feel good and have fun, bringing your life into better balance. If you're afraid to let go of old habits, remember: the person who is able to control his working life is more likely to be good at the job.

Creative leisure
Creative leisure uses your 'inner child' who longs to enjoy, to be playful and to take risks. To give your inner child a chance to speak and decide on what it wants to do is to become a more complete and contented person.

Have you ever thought of going to a painting or writing class, or making pottery? You don't have to be good at it, the best in the class – you just need to give it attention and enjoy it.

Physical skills – horse-riding, scuba diving – can give you a tremendous thrill. If you prefer something quieter (and cheaper) there are evening classes available in everything, from lace-making to languages.

If your work involves long hours in front of a screen, try a contrasting spare-time activity that uses your body to the full – sport, dance, or just peaceful walking in the country.

> **If your work involves long hours in front of a screen, try a contrasting spare-time activity that uses your body to the full**

Perhaps your job demands split-second decisions for which you are entirely responsible. In that case, choose a leisure pursuit where you give the onus to someone else; help to crew a yacht, perhaps, or lend a hand with a local theatre group.

Is your job dull, with little mental stimulus? You could attend lectures on literature, art – anything that interests you and opens doors into greater appreciation and knowledge of the subject.

All these activities bring greater self-confidence with them as you enlarge your world and learn to understand new things.

Change your priorities

Has your work pattern cut you off from the people you love? Try giving family, lover, friends, a little more time; you (and they) will be delighted at the attention and affection which have been given second place for so long.

Do you enjoy helping others? There's a huge network of people in your neighbourhood who devote a few hours each week to making life pleasanter for somebody else. Your local library will put you in the picture.

Looking after yourself

Have you forgotten how to unwind? See the Stress and Fatigue chapter for advice on rapid and effective ways to relax.

DOWNSHIFTING

Some people are now making radical changes to the way they earn their money and organise their lives. This downshifting is a response to the intense pressures of modern working life, with its disillusionments and uncertainties.

Downshifting usually means working less hard (and earning less) so that you have more time to enjoy your life. But it can also mean the start of a new, self-employed career, just as demanding but infinitely more rewarding than the old one.

WHY DO PEOPLE DOWNSHIFT?

According to a 1994 Gallup poll, a third of all Americans would be willing to take a 20 per cent cut in income if they or their partner could work fewer hours. An international survey of 1,300 executives found that two-thirds put their family, health and outside interests above money.

People are coming home from work too tired to take pleasure in their private lives. Almost half the British workforce feels absolutely exhausted after work, compared with 36 per cent in the US and 17 per cent in Holland. The inability to enjoy life after work is an international problem.

Many marriages barely survive the pressures of work, and many children only see their parents at weekends because Mum or Dad are busy and constantly have to employ babysitters.

No longer can we count on the same job for life. With changes in the workplace and economic downturns bringing compulsory redundancies, flexibility and adaptability are the key now.

Says business psychologist John Nicholson, 'The man or woman who does not seek the trappings of a large corporation around them, who is willing to build a niche in the market, and to change careers several times during the course of their working lives, will flourish in this decentralised world. Small will be beautiful, believe me.'

HOW TO DOWNSHIFT

Is downshifting for you?

If you have a huge mortgage and many other family expenses which you can't jettison, then downshifting is not an option.

Changing your life can mean small changes or big upheavals.

- Can you cope with change?
- Do you enjoy the idea of a new start, a fresh challenge?
- Are you ready to take on the risks as well as the highs?
- Can you find satisfaction for yourself and your family in a lifestyle that does not include constant, high-level spending?

- Can you increase activities – country walks, galleries and museums, picnics, joining local societies – that cost little or nothing?

> *There are few activities more energising and rejuvenating than taking charge of your own working life and changing it to suit yourself*

If you have always worked for a large corporation you may find the idea of striking out on your own in a search for less exhausting, more fulfilling work rather alarming. Can you ride this stage for the sake of your future?

If you do decide to downshift, you will discover that there are few activities more energising and rejuvenating than taking charge of your own working life and changing it to suit yourself.

Before starting, you must be clear about your plans:
- What do you want from this change?
- How radical do you want the change to be?
- How do you plan on getting what you want?
- What is the minimum income you need to get by?
- What do you have behind you in the bank for emergencies?
- What are your family commitments?
- What are your skills, training, experience?
- What are your contacts, i.e. friends and colleagues who can offer work?
- What are your strengths?

These need to include:
- keeping going in the face of disappointment and uncertainty
- handling money without getting into debt or overspending

- being flexible and adaptable about both your working life and your new spare time
- being patient and self-disciplined
- putting in enough work to realise your goals
- coping with new challenges on your own

What are the possibilities? Could you ask your employers if they would let you job-share or work fewer hours? Can you find part-time work which allows you more spare time?

Betty, a 45-year-old widow, now works part-time as a legal secretary. She has let a room in her large house to a student, and finds she has more time for friends and family.

Tax consultant George now works almost all the time from home, using his PC. Self-employed, George draws on years of experience in dealing with the Inland Revenue to help a growing circle of clients.

Ann took the plunge and left inner-city teaching altogether, feeling disillusioned and burnt out. She used her savings – and occasionally her husband's income – to help her train in complementary medicine and now runs a flourishing practice as an acupuncturist. 'I don't work nine to five any more,' she says, 'but I do make enough to enjoy life – and I don't have to lean on my husband for money any more. Work varies from week to week, but I've learned to accept this and not worry about it. You need to be completely self-motivated in this field.'

If you want to free yourself from a vicious circle of overwork and overspending, with its disillusionment and fatigue, downshifting may be for you.

For more information
Read: *Downshifting: The Ultimate Handbook* by Andy Bull (Thorsons, 1998).

CHAPTER 17

Energy and Your Home

What does your home mean to you?

For some of us, it's just a place where we sleep and leave our things. For others (perhaps the majority) it's a place where we can rest, feel secure and recharge our batteries in a familiar environment that reflects the sort of people we are.

For most people a home is a vital part of life, a centre where we can enjoy solitude and think things over, meet with the people we love and find new energies for tomorrow.

This peaceful unwinding, this process of self-nourishment, is an art that many high-flyers depend on: the ability to switch off, to take refuge. If you have a young family, home can be a place where you enjoy and encourage them. For you and your partner, home is probably the only place where you can be really alone together.

Primitive peoples believed that every home had its spirits protecting it and they would put food out at night for their guardians. In ancient Rome, food spilled on the floor was left for a while until the domestic spirits had taken their share.

It's very easy nowadays to forget home, to cease to tend this special haven in our rushed lives, to forgo the pleasure we can get from simply pottering: reading, listening to music, gossiping with friends and family, watering the plants or just watching TV. But this relaxing, recharging process has a tremendous impact on our attitudes and appetite for life.

So we need to be aware of what our homes can give us in

terms of the peace and repose that bring with them increased energy and better health.

You can if you wish spend vast amounts of money and time on improving your home – there are plenty of books and magazines to give you ideas. But what's really vital is that it's right for you, a place which you and your family will enjoy and which makes you feel good every time you come through the front door. It's an atmosphere, created by attractive lighting, comfortable places to sit, and harmonious colours, scents and sounds. If you're a genius with the needle or DIY, you can create much of this beauty yourself. If not, careful choices and planning can buy it for you, without breaking the bank.

CLUTTER

An elderly friend of mine, a retired professor, lives in a tiny house literally crammed with heaped-up back copies of the *Financial Times* – on the floor, on the chairs, on the windowsills, everywhere. 'Don't touch anything,' he will say, lovingly clutching a faded edition from 1942, 'I might need it.'

Absent-minded professors have their own rules but, for most of us, it's hard to feel clear-headed and at ease in a room piled high with clutter. It seems that all those newspapers, magazines, coffee cups, buttons, old shopping lists, are all silently waiting to be dealt with, in mute reproach, and this saps our energies, making us feel muddled and indecisive. So, cut down your clutter.

If it's painful to throw away things that are linked to the past but completely useless in the present, do it in small stages. Clear out a magazine rack one day, perhaps, and a store cupboard the next. If you throw away the old cardigan that Aunt Dora used to

For most of us, it's hard to feel clear-headed and at ease in a room piled high with clutter

wear before she died, don't worry; she won't mind.

You'll be amazed at the lifting of spirits that an uncluttered house will give you.

DIRT

Keep your home clean. Aim to keep down the dirt and untidiness with as little hassle as possible. Work out a system for cleaning (to include your family!). Your get-out clause is severe rush or overwork, when forcing yourself to run around cleaning will result in frayed nerves and dropped cups. Home doesn't have to be so perfect that people are afraid to breathe or walk on the floor, but it does have to be clean enough to make you feel good.

SPACE

Space is something we all need, a quality in our lives which, when it's lacking, can cause tiredness, irritability and sometimes even panic.

A woman acquaintance of mine was an enthusiastic photographer; so enthusiastic, in fact, that she gave her home over completely to piles of photographs and mounds of assorted equipment. Her unfortunate husband had barely any space to himself. He ended up an alcoholic. Was there a connection?

Everyone needs a space they can call their own, and the best place for this is at home.

HOME AND YOUR SENSES

Colour

Colour is a vital part of our lives which we take for granted; we give little conscious thought to the effects that the blue of water and sky, the green of plants and the countless other colours and shades of our world have upon us. Research has found that different colours work in different ways on our nervous system and feelings – for example, people in a blue room tend to feel chillier than

> *Different colours work in different ways on our nervous system and feelings*

those in a red room – and your choice of colours says a great deal about the kind of person you are. Colour in the home is of major importance.

Here's what colour does:

Red: Linked with power, energy and courage, red can actually increase your pulse and breathing rate and stimulate your brain. Red wakes you up, so it's not a good colour for bedrooms and should not be used in a room where you stay for long periods. It makes dark passages, however, look warm and inviting.

Orange: This colour also creates energy, and makes you feel confident and friendly. It is ideal for a dining room (it can make people feel hungry!) or a living room.

Yellow: Another colour to lift the spirits and increase energy, yellow can give you confidence, stimulate the logical, clear-thinking part of your brain and improve your memory. You might paint your kitchen yellow.

Green: A restful, cool colour which can soothe and ease stress.

Blue: Another cool, soothing natural colour, blue also encourages communication and clear thinking.

Indigo (midnight blue):   Said to restore emotional balance, calming indigo would look good in a bedroom.

Violet: Gentle violet soothes body and mind and can help with anxiety and insomnia.

White: Clear and calming. If used in large blocks, it serves best as a background to small patches of other, vivid colours.

Brown: Increasingly popular, earthy brown is the third natural colour, richly warm, reassuring and strong.

Black: Marvellous in small doses, black is believed to heighten emotional response.

Neutral shades: Ever-popular, cream and off-white are good relaxing background colours for the home, but grey can be depressing.

You can use colour to change your home dramatically without spending a fortune. If you make a terrible mistake you can always paint over it! It's how a colour makes *you* feel that matters – so, to change your mood and energy levels, the choice is yours.

Sound

Do you like sound in your home? Background music can be very pleasant, but some people prefer tranquil silence, particularly if their working lives are spent under a constant barrage of sound – machinery, traffic, canned music – which can disrupt concentration, fray nerves and drain away energy. Soft, slow music will soothe you, and loud music with an insistent beat will stimulate, as will anything emotional or witty. You may find familiar everyday sounds – the distant hum of traffic, the coo of pigeons, gentle talk in the garden – reassuring and peaceful.

Smell

Flowers, pot-pourri and scented candles add another pleasant dimension: the sense of smell. Don't be ashamed of cooking odours; why spray your kitchen with aerosol chemicals when it smells so appetising? Essential oils, sprinkled over pot-pourri or in a burner, add delicious scents; lavender, Roman camomile, clary sage or neroli are calming, and rosemary, pine and citrus oils such as lemon are energisers.

PROTECTING YOUR HOME

The modern home contains many pollutants which can cause fatigue and illness in vulnerable people. Here's how to make it a safer place to live in.

CHEMICALS

When they are new, synthetic carpets give off organic compounds such as formaldehyde, a common chemical also used on curtains, wood furniture and walls and found in some clothes, drugs, cosmetics, shampoos and perfumes. In sensitive people formaldehyde can cause allergic reactions including flu-like symptoms.

Other common household chemicals that make some people ill are found in:

- insect and polish sprays
- other aerosols
- adhesives
- wood preservatives
- paints
- paint solvents
- cleaners
- many plastic products

To reduce the effects of these chemicals, open the windows after you have used them and immediately after you have had synthetic carpets fitted.

Carpets made of wool, cotton, sisal, jute, seagrass or coir are safe and readily available now, as are cleaners and many other household products made from natural substances.

AIR

Carbon monoxide (CO) is a poisonous gas produced when gas, wood or coal is used for cooking and heating; it has no smell, taste or colour and, if allowed to leak into the air, causes fatigue, headaches, nausea and dizziness and can even kill. See your appliances are serviced regularly. (CO detectors are also available.)

Tobacco smoke is a well-recognised hazard so, if you have a smoker in the house, make sure your home is well ventilated; this will also hinder infections from spreading round the family.

Plants can clear your house of chemical fumes. Particularly good, according to Jane Alexander in her book *Spirit of the Home* (Thorsons, 1998) are:

> *Plants can clear your house of chemical fumes*

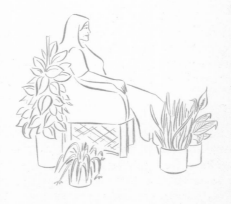

- peace lilies
- dwarf banana plants
- golden pothos
- peperomias
- spider plants
- mother-in-law's tongue
- Chinese evergreens
- goosefoot plants

Negative ions are natural molecules created by sunlight and thunderstorms which clean up the air, destroying airborne bacteria and clearing the atmosphere of dust, pollen and smoke. Ionisers are small portable boxes which emit negative ions, helpful for headaches, depression and fatigue (and often allergies and breathing problems, too). Electronic equipment, stale air and static all reduce negative ions, so place your ioniser near your computer or TV set (see the end of the chapter for supplier).

Radon gas can seep into houses from the domestic water system, causing flu-like symptoms. If you are aware of a local problem, contact your environmental health officer for help.

LIGHT

Let in as much natural light as you can; see Energy from Nature for more details. Of all the types of artificial lighting, fluorescent is the worst for health; tungsten is better; and full-spectrum lighting the best (see the end of the chapter for supplier).

WATER

Your tapwater is not necessarily pure. It may contain agricultural chemicals and toxic metals, and the chemicals added to it can also upset some people.

Bottled waters usually taste better than water straight from the tap, but they're not always chemical-free. A jug filter is the cheapest and simplest way to purify your water to some extent (removing chlorine, pesticides and herbicides) although jug filters do not usually remove fluoride or agricultural nitrates; expensive plumbed-in filters can do this. (Fluoride is controversial and its benefits debatable. Fluoride overload is linked with fatigue, indigestion, muscular and joint pains and skin symptoms.) With a jug filter, always be careful to change the cartridge regularly; an overloaded cartridge will 'dump' the pollutants back into the water again.

Plumbed-in filters remove more pollutants but cost more as well.

EMF

Modern, high-tech living surrounds us with electromagnetic fields. It's been estimated that our bodies now have to deal with up to 200 million times more electromagnetic signals than those of our ancestors. At home, we have radio and TV waves, microwaves, night-storage heaters and a host of other electronic equipment.

Electromagnetic stress can cause fatigue, depression, headaches and many other symptoms.

Always switch off the TV or computer when you're not using it. Laptops are safer, with their crystal displays, but all the same don't work with one actually on your lap.

Don't fall asleep in front of the television and don't allow children to sit right up against it. Use an old-fashioned hot water bottle instead of an electric blanket and site your bed away from night-storage heaters.

For more information
Ionisers: Contact the Wholistic Research Company at The Old Forge, Mill Green, Hatfield, Hertfordshire AL9 5NZ; telephone 01707 262686; fax 01707 258828.

Full-spectrum lighting: Contact FSL at 19 Lincoln Road, Cressex Business Park, High Wycombe, Bucks HP12 3FX; telephone 014945 26051.

CHAPTER 18

Finding a Qualified Practitioner

Many local libraries carry practitioner lists.

Acupuncture

For details of your local practitioners, send a 9″ × 6″ sae to the British Acupuncture Council, 63 Jeddo Road, London W12 9HQ; telephone 020 8735 0400; website www.acupuncture.org.uk.

Medical Herbalism

For details of your local practitioners, send a 9″ × 6″ sae with two first-class stamps to the International Register of Consultant Herbalists, 32 King Edward's Road, Swansea SA1 4LL; telephone 01792 655886; website www.irch.org.

Homeopathy

For a list of medically qualified practitioners, write to the British Homoeopathic Association, 15 Clerkenwell Close, London EC1R 0AA; telephone 020 7566 7800.

For a list of lay practitioners, send an sae to the Society of Homoeopaths, 4A Artisan Road, Northampton NN1 4HU; telephone 01604 621400; website www.homoeopathy.org.uk.

Naturopathy (and Osteopathy)

For a list of practitioners, send a cheque for £2.50 to the General Council and Register of Naturopaths, Goswell House, 2 Goswell Road, Street, Somerset BA16 0JG; telephone 01458 840072; website www.naturopathy.org.uk.

Nutrition

Many practitioners offer nutritional advice. For a register of nutritionists, however, send a cheque for £2.00 to the Institute for Optimum Nutrition, Blades Court, Deodar Road, London SW15 2NU, or, for a local practitioner, call the ION on 020 8877 9993.

Yoga

Visit your local library for a list of classes, or contact the Yoga Therapy Centre, Homeopathic Hospital, 60 Great Ormond Street, London WC1N 3HR; telephone 020 7419 7195; website www.yogatherapy.org.